Ketogenic Diet for Weight Loss

A Keto Diet Plan With Enticing Ketogenic Diet Recipes!

William Brownie

Table-Of-Contents

Introduction

At first, the world was skeptical. Who could blame it? The Ketogenic Diet turned the ingrained wisdom of 'proper' nutrition, not to mention the sacred food pyramid, on it's head. Eat more fat, it proudly proclaimed, and you will lose all the fat you need.

It seemed ridiculous. Unhealthy. Death dealing.

Twenty years down the track, the skeptics are few and far between. A mountain of scientific evidence now supports the ketogenic diet as, not only the most effective fat loss method that exists, but also one of the healthiest. That's great news for food lovers. After all, fat is what gives food its flavor.

This book celebrates the love of food. We have embraced the freedom of more fat to produce truly mouth-watering fare. The recipes to follow not only meet your low carb requirement, but also engage your taste buds with a range of flavors, textures and visual appeal that will have you scarcely believing that what you're eating is good for you.

Chapter 1: Ketogenic Diet Basics

What is the Ketogenic Diet?

The ketogenic diet is a high fat, moderate protein, low carb diet designed to force the body to switch from using glucose from carbohydrates to using ketones from fat as its primary energy source. It does this by restricting the intake of carbohydrates and increasing the amount of fat consumed.

The word ketogenesis means that we burn fat as our energy supply. When fatty acids are broken down they become ketones. The body can either use glucose or ketones to produce adenosine triphosphate (ATP), which is the body's energy source. Without ATP, we would not be alive. Everything we do is dependent on it.

When we take carbohydrates into our body, it ends up as glucose. The body uses glucose to burn energy and become ATP. When we consume protein, it is broken down into amino acids. Amino acids build and maintain the body. When we ingest fats, they become ketones. Ketones also have the ability to produce ATP. The goal of the ketogenic diet is to only use fats as the body's energy source.

The ketogenic diet mimics the effects of fasting. In a fasted state the body produces ketones, as a result of the body having to burn stored fat rather carbohydrates. The original ketogenic diet had a fat to protein and carbs ratio of 4 to 1.

Keto Means No More Cravings

The meals that you eat on the ketogenic diet are extremely satisfying and nutritious. They will fill you up, meaning that you'll have fewer cravings and experience less time when you are hungry. That's because it is fat that triggers satiation, or the feeling of fullness.

When you are in a state of ketosis, your body will burn the fat that it has already stored as a means of energy. What's more, it will do so without the extra release of insulin that accompanies carbohydrate intake. You thus avoid the blood sugar highs and crashes that come with eating carb foods.

Keto Diet History

Despite its recent surge in popularity, the ketogenic diet has been around for a long time. It was originally developed in 1924 by Dr. Russell Wilder of the Mayo Clinic. Dr. Wilder was looking for a way to treat epileptic children who weren't responding to normal medication. His ketogenic diet worked wonders.

However, with the advent of new powerful anti-seizure drugs, and the influence of drug companies, the ketogenic diet for treating juvenile epilepsy fell out of favor.

The modern keto revival began in 1994, when Charlie Abrahams, the son of Hollywood director John Abrahams was successfully treated with the diet. There followed a lot of media exposure, including a popular movie called First Do No Harm, starring Meryl

Streep, about the treatment of a child's intractable epilepsy with the keto diet.

The publicity revolving around the keto diet's benefits in treating epilepsy led to studies to determine if it could also benefit the people in general. There is now a body of research showing that the keto diet is a successful and safe route to rapid fat loss.

Is It Safe?

Yes. The keto diet has been the subject of a large number of studies that have shown that it is a safe way to lose body fat. Many of the concerns over the diet are the result of long-standing misunderstandings about fat and the role it plays in our health. The truth is that fat will not make you fat. Neither will it ruin your cardiovascular health. Too many carbohydrates will both make you fat and unhealthy. That is why the keto diet cuts out carbs.

How is the Keto Diet Different than Other Diet Plans

The Keto takes most other diet plans and stands them on their head. The common denominator of the majority of diets is restricted fat intake. With the keto diet, your goal is to eat more saturated fat.

Traditional diets almost universally encourage increased fruit and vegetable consumption. The keto diet cuts out the majority of vegetables and fruits, but does allow for a generous amount of green, starchy vegetables such as lettuce and spinach.
Traditional diets are built around caloric restriction. On the keto diet, this is not necessary.

Most diets generally follow the Food Guide Pyramid model. The keto diet does the opposite. The foods that form the base of the Food Guide Pyramid, whole grains, are eliminated from the keto diet, while those at the top, saturated fats, are encouraged.

On the majority of other diets, restricted caloric intake leads to cravings, constant hunger and, possibly, binging. On the keto diet, you do not experience any of those effects. Because you are mainly eating saturated fats, you will feel full and satisfied after your meals. There will be no urge to snack between meals and no chances of falling off the diet wagon.

Many diet plans require the user to purchase expensive meal products from the organization behind the diet. There is none of this with the Keto diet.

How Does the Keto Diet Differ from the Atkins Diet?

The popularity of low carb dieting can largely be attributed to Dr. Robert Atkins, with his book The Diet Revolution in 1972. At first glance, the ketogenic diet looks very similar to the Atkins diet. There are, however some key differences:

On Atkins you can eat as much protein as you like, whereas on a keto diet you have to moderate your protein intake. The reason is that there is a process known as gluconeogenesis, by where the body will convert excess protein to glucose. This defeats the purpose of going low carb, as your blood stream will be filled with just as much glucose as when you were eating high carb.

On Atkins, you start with zero carbs and, therefore, put yourself in a ketogenic state (though Dr. Atkins never actually used the term 'ketogenic'). This is known as the induction phase of the Atkins program. From there, carbs are slowly reintroduced to the diet. With the keto diet, you do not re-introduce carbs.

With Atkins, you go through a number of phases: Induction, Ongoing Weight Loss, Pre-maintenance, Lifetime maintenance. At each stage you manipulate your carb intake. There are no such phases on the keto diet.

How Does the Keto Diet Differ from the Paleo Diet?

Both Paleo and Keto are low carb. However, whereas the Keto diet is built around manipulating your macro nutrient intake (high fat, moderate protein, low carb), the focus of the Paleo diet is on food choices. With Paleo you cut out dairy products, grains and processed foods. The low carb diet that results is a consequence of this process, not the goal in itself. With the remaining foods that you do eat, there is no emphasis on restricting carbs.

The Paleo Diet is also known as The Caveman Diet, The Stone Age Diet and the New Evolutionary Diet. It is a modern day attempt to emulate the eating habits of Paleolithic humans. The Paleolithic period lasted from some 2.5 million years ago until the start of the agricultural age, which began around 8,000 CE. During that period of time people ate what they were able to hunt, kill and gather. That means that their diet was high in . . .

> ➢ Wild game
> ➢ Fish
> ➢ Nuts and seeds
> ➢ Green leafy vegetables,

➢ Root vegetables
➢ Fruit
➢ Berries

The Paleo Diet, then, is composed of a simple maxim:

Eat what our cave dwelling ancestors ate and stay away from what he didn't eat

With Paleo, there is no attempt to enter into the state of ketogenesis.

Why It Is Important to Visit Your Doctor on a Regular Basis?

The ketogenic diet is a specialized eating lifestyle. It designed to make you healthier, lose body fat and promote general well being. Visiting with your doctor to inform him of your intention to follow the diet is a smart decision.

There have a been a huge number of studies that have confirmed the powerful effects of the Keto diet in terms of fat loss and health enhancement. Most doctors will be aware of them. However, the majority of general practitioners are not trained nutritionists. Some doctors may express concerns between the desired state of ketosis and the condition known as ketoacidosis. Ketoacidosis is a rare life threatening condition that can occur in Type-1 diabetics.

Your doctor will quite properly advise you not to follow a ketogenic diet if you are:

> A Type-1 diabetic
> Primary Carnitine deficient
> Carnitine translocase deficient
> Beta-oxidation defective
> Suffering from impaired liver function
> Suffering from gall bladder disease
> A gastric bypass surgery recipient
> Plagued with abnormal tumors
> Pregnant or breastfeeding

You should have regular check ups and blood tests while you are on the ketogenic diet. These will allow you to monitor your progress in terms of not just fat loss, which you can readily see, but your vital cardio health markers as well. This will provide you with on going motivation and peace of mind as you see the raw data that eating more fat is not increasing your cholesterol and blood pressure levels but is, in fact, bringing them down.

Chapter 2: Advantages of the Ketogenic Diet

The ketogenic diet is ideal for fat loss, Type 2 diabetes, cancer and neurological diseases. Here are the top 10 benefits of going on the ketogenic diet.

1) Losing Weight.

When you go on the ketogenic diet you are going to lose weight in the form of body fat. You will starve your body so much of carbs, that it is being forced to burn fat to supply the ATP that your body needs. As a result, you will burn fat 24/7.

When you eat a lot of sugar, your body holds on to sodium. As a result, your kidneys don't work as effectively. You won't urinate enough and your body will store waste products. Switch to a keto diet, and your kidneys will work so much more efficiently. You body will flush out your system. As a result, you will lose weight. (1)

2)Treating Type 2 Diabetes

Type 2 diabetics are people who have lost their insulin sensitivity. When you are insulin sensitive, your cells will absorb only the carbs that insulin tells it to. Nut when you eat so any carbs that you become insulin sensitive, the cells don't react to insulin any more. However, when you go on a ketogenic diet, you starve yourself of sugar. Your body releases more and more ketones as an alternative form of fuel. As a result, your insulin sensitivity will go back to normal.

Although we do not recommend the ketogenic diet for people who are diabetic, it is ideal for those who are pre-diabetic. People with full-blown diabetes will produce too many ketones and get into diabetic acidosis, which is very dangerous.

For people who are pre-diabetic, however, the carb restriction will quickly reverse their insulin resistance. (2)

3)Cancer Treatment

The Ketogenic diet has been seen to be extremely beneficial for the treatment of cancer. It is known that cancerous cells feed off sugar. When you deplete sugar from your system, the cancer cells no longer have an energy source. These cells will die and the cancer will decrease. (3)

4)Combatting Neurological Diseases

The Ketogenic diet is an effective fighter against neurological diseases. Such conditions as depression, anxiety, Alzheimer's disease, Parkinson's disease, dementia, can all be positively treated with this diet. When you produce more ketones and less glucose, our bodies experience less oxidative stress. Oxidative stress is bad for our brain health and produces inflammation. The keto diet is also believed to cause the mitochondria within the cells to work more effectively. In some neurological diseases, the mitochondrial process has been disoriented. The reduced sugar of the keto diet helps to rebalance this mitochondrial activity. (4)

5) Appetite Suppressant

The keto diet kills your appetite. When you eat very low carb, you don't get hungry because you are supplementing your sugar with fat. Studies show that when lowering carbs to enter ketosis while eating more fat and protein, you eat fewer calories. (5)

6) Losing Visceral Body Fat

On a keto diet you will lose more visceral abdominal fat. Visceral fat smothers your vital organs, preventing them from working efficiently. When you are on a high fat / low carb diet plan, your body will shed that visceral fat. (6)

7) Reduces Triglycerides

The keto diet will reduce the levels of triglycerides in your bloodstream. High triglycerides area result of eating too much sugar. High fructose corn syrup is the main culprit. On the keto diet you won't be having any of it! (7)

8)Increases Good Cholesterol

The keto diet increases the proportion of HDL cholesterol in the body. There are two types of cholesterol in your system, high density (HDL) and low density (LDL) lipoproteins. They both act like taxi cabs, transporting cholesterol around the body. Whereas LDL transports the cholesterol to your organs, HDL takes it away from them and delivers it to the liver for use as energy or excretion. The best way to increase the levels of HDH is to eat high fat. (8)

9)Fights Metabolic Syndrome

The keto diet fights metabolic syndrome. Metabolic syndrome is a collective term for the following symptoms:
> Abdominal obesity
> Elevated blood pressure
> Elevated blood sugar levels
> Elevated triglycerides
> Low HDL

All of these areas will be drastically improved on the keto diet. (9)

10) Provides More Energy

You will feel full of energy on the keto diet. You will rid yourself of fatigue, you will experience more clarity, feeling more alert and wide awake. You will even sleep better when you follow the keto diet. (10)

Chapter 3: Food Guidelines

The Macronutrients

Protein

Protein is the building material of the body. Everything is made from it, from your hair to your toe nails. Protein is made up of amino acids, which join together like the carriages of a train to build different parts of you.

Of the three macronutrients, protein is the most satiating, and carbohydrate is the least satiating. That means that protein will fill you up faster. Protein also burns more calories in the process of digestion.

A key protein consideration when eating for low carbs is the state of gluconeogenesis. This is the process by which your body is able to make glucose from non-carbohydrate sources, including protein. In the absence of carbs in the diet, the body will look to convert protein into glucose. If there is insufficient protein in the diet, it will take protein from your muscle tissue and use it for energy. However, if there is too much protein coursing through the body, the unused portion will be converted to glucose. This will fight against your efforts to attain to a ketogenic state.

For these reasons it is very important that you don't take in either too little or too much protein.

So, just how much protein should you be taking in? That depends on your activity level. If you are exercising regularly, especially if you are a weight trainer, you will need more protein than in you are sedentary.

To work out your protein range, simply multiply your weight in pounds by 0.6 and 1.0 to provide your range. So, if you are 180 pounds, your range would be:

$$0.6 \times 180 = 108$$

$$1.0 \quad \times 180 = 180$$

So, the range would be 108-180 grams per day. If you are a sedentary person, you would go with 108 grams. A hard training weight lifter would take in 180 grams of protein per day.

Best Protein Sources

- Eggs
- Chicken breast
- Beef
- Fish
- Pork
- Whey Protein Powder
- Cheese
- Soy

Fat

There are three different types of fat in our food:

- **Saturated Fat** – For decades they've been seen as the enemy to good health, but recent studies have shown that saturated fats actually promote immune system health, balance testosterone levels and increase bone density. The belief that they are linked to heart disease has also been shown to be a myth. Get your saturated fats from:

  - ✓ Eggs
  - ✓ Butter
  - ✓ Meat

- **Polyunsaturated Fat** – The most common forms of polyunsaturated fats are vegetable oils. For a long time we've been told that they are good for us. However, the majority of them are highly processed. Processed polyunsaturated are not good for you and should be avoided.

An essential fatty acid is one that your body needs but can't assemble from other fats. You have to get it whole, from foods. The two key essential fatty acids (EFA's) are . . .

- ✓ Omega -3 (alpha linolenic – LNA)
- ✓ Omega-6 (linolenic – LA)

The typical diet is rich in omega-6 fatty acids, but not in omega-3. In fact, the average person takes in 20 times more omega-6 than they do omega-3. One reason for this huge disparity is the huge amount of refined grains compared with the miniscule amount of fatty fish and other onega-3 rich foods that we tend to consume.

Here are some benefits of increasing your intake of Omega-3 Fatty Acids:

- ✓ Improved insulin sensitivity

- ✓ Better absorption of fat-soluble vitamins
- ✓ Improved joint health
- ✓ Enhanced energy
- ✓ Better oxygen transfer
- ✓ Enhanced cell membrane integrity
- ✓ Better suppression of cortisol
- ✓ Improved skin texture
- ✓ Promotes muscle growth
- ✓ Increases your metabolism
- ✓ Helps burn fat

Add these foods to your diet to boost your intake of healthy fats:

- ✓ Fatty Fish (salmon, tuna)
- ✓ Flax seed Oil
- ✓ Coconut Oil
- ✓ Avocado
- ✓ Nuts and Seeds

➢ **Trans Fats** - Trans fats are created when vegetable oil goes under a process known as hydrogenation. This is done to extend the shelf life of the food. Trans fats are commonly found in commercially fried foods, cookies, margarines and crackers.

The hydrogenation process makes vegetable oils act like saturated fats. They raise the levels of LDL cholesterol, lading to an increased risk of heart disease.

To avoid trans fats opt for coconut, hemp, olive or sesame oil.

80% of your macronutrients should come in the form of fats on the keto diet.

Carbohydrates

Though you will be going very low on carbs, you won't be cutting out altogether. One reason is that a small amount of carbs will prevent the body from burning protein for energy. In addition, non-starchy carbs contain vital fiber which we need to function properly. So, while you should avoid all starchy carbs like peas, potatoes, corn and squash, you can and should eat the following:

> - Any leafy green vegetable
> - Alfalfa sprouts
> - Avocado
> - Brussels sprouts
> - Cabbage
> - Carrots

> ➢ Kale
> ➢ Mushrooms
> ➢ Turnips

Total and Net Carbs

Fiber is a form of carbohydrate that contains molecules that are much bigger than other carbs. In fact, they are so big that they cannot be digested by the body and pass through your body without being absorbed. As a result, fibrous carbs will not push up your blood sugar levels or lead to the release of insulin.

Fibrous carbs will, in fact, help to slow down the absorption of starches and sugars. They are, therefore, a valuable addition to your diet. That is why we will subtract the number of fibrous carbs when working out your caloric totals. The carb count including fiber will be referred to as the amount of total carbs. The total with fiber removed we will call the net carbs. It is the net carbs that we need to keep as low as possible.

Calorie Counting

For the first few weeks of your transition to the keto diet, you will need to count your calories. However, this is more to ensure that you stay within your macronutrient levels than total caloric content. The most important macronutrient number, of course, is you total daily net carbs.

Carbs should make up just 2.5% of your daily caloric total. That means that, if you are taking in 2000 calories per day, your total carbs will be 50 calories.

Fats will comprise 80% of your caloric intake. On a 2000 calorie diet, that equates to 1,600 calories.

That leaves 17.5% to come from protein. On 2000 calories per day, you'd be taking in 350 calories from protein each day.

Measuring your food will require the following items:

- ✓ A food diary
- ✓ A set of food scales
- ✓ A set of measuring cups

You may also wish to invest in an App that will calculate your calories and macros for you. Here are a couple of options that will make your life so much easier:

https://www.loseit.com/

http://www.sparkpeople.com/index2.asp

Finding Your Daily Caloric Level

In order to work out what your personal macro numbers are, you need to fist establish what your daily caloric requirements are. To do that you need to know about two things:

BMR = Basal Metabolic Rate is the number of calories that you need each day to stay alive at your current weight. If you were lying in bed all day, it would be the number of calories you needed to function. To work out your BMR use the following formula . . .

BMR = 10 x weight (kg) + 6.25 x height (cm) - 5 x 22 + 5

> ➢ 1 inch=2.54cm
> ➢ 1lb =.453592 kg

TDEE = Total Daily Energy Expenditure is your BMR plus the extra calories that you use up throughout your daily activities. TDEE allocates calories in accordance with the following activity groupings:

> ➢ Sedentary - desk job, very little exercise
> ➢ Slight Activity- light exercise, one to three days per week
> ➢ Moderate Activity- moderate exercise, three to five days per week
> ➢ Very Active - hard exercise, six to seven days per week
> ➢ Extreme Activity - hard daily exercise plus a job that is physical

To calculate your TDEE, you multiply your BMR by a factor based upon activity grouping. The factors are:

> ➢ Sedentary - 1.2
> ➢ Slight Activity - 1.3
> ➢ Moderate Activity - 1.5
> ➢ Very Active - 1.7

Let's take a look at an example to see how we can work out total calories and macronutrient levels.

Steve is 32 years old and 90 kg. He is 180 cm tall. He trains 5 days per week on a heavy, compound exercise based program. He's a teacher who spends most of his day at the front of a classroom.

Steve belongs on the Moderate Activity Level of the TDEE activity scale. This gives him at TDEE factor of 1.5.

We now have to work out Steve's BMR using our formula . . .

BMR = 10 x weight (kg) + 6.25 x height (cm) - 5 x 22 + 5

10 x 90 + (6.25 x 180) - (5 x 22) + 5

1920

We can now work out Steve's TDEE by multiplying his BMR by 1.5 BMR = 10 x weight (kg) + 6.25 x height (cm) - 5 x 22 + 5

1920 x 1.5 = 2880

In order to maintain his current body weight, Steve needs to take in 2880 calories per day. But we want him to lose body fat not stay the same. Our goal is to drop one pound of fat through nutrition every single week. To do that we will set his daily caloric total 500 calories lower than his TDEE.

2880 - 500 = 2380

We now have Steve's total daily caloric total: 2380

Steve's macronutrient levels would be:
  ➢ Fat = 1904 calories
  ➢ Protein = 416 calories

There are 9 calories in 1 gram of fat.
There are 4 calories in 1 gram of protein and carbohydrate.

We can use these numbers to work out Steve's macro intake in terms of grams of food.

Fat = 1904 / 9 = 212 grams
Protein = 416 / 4 = 104 grams
Carbs = 60/4 = 15 grams

Nine Low Carb Baking Substitutions

Flour, an essential baking ingredient, is a high carb food. Fortunately, there are plenty of low carb substitutes available that will allow you to produce baking delicacies without blowing out your carb count. Here are 9 alternatives that will give you the freedom to bake to your heart's delight, knowing that the treats you're pulling from the oven are low carb.

Coconut Flour

Coconut flour is completely sugar free. It's protein rich and full of fiber. Rather than producing a coconut rich flavor to your baked goods, it will remind you more of vanilla pound cake. The high fiber content makes it very filling. Plus, it's gluten free. And, because it absorbs a lot of water, you only need 1/3 as much flour as the recipe calls for.
Coconut flour is great for making:

- ✓ Pancakes
- ✓ Quick bread
- ✓ Cakes

Almond Flour

Although containing more fat than coconut flour, almond flour will result in a baked product that is moist and tender. It is made from ground almonds, giving a high protein content. However, it's quite a bit more expensive than coconut flour

Protein Powder

Yes, that whey powder that you put into your shake is also an excellent replacement for sugar. Good protein powders will contain an emulsifier which will readily absorb liquids. Look for powders that contain no artificial colors or flavorings.

Pumpkin Puree

Pumpkin puree can do a great job as a replacement for high carb fruits or other ingredients, resulting in a moist end product. You can also use it to replace bananas, which are high in carbs. It goes great with coconut flour.

Apple Sauce

Use apple sauce to replace oils and sweeteners in recipes. It's low in sugar and allows you to use fewer eggs in your recipes.

Stevia

Stevia should become your 'go to' sweetener. It's completely natural, actually reduces blood sugar levels and is stronger than sugar, so you need less of it. It is available in liquid or powdered form. Just make that the version you buy doesn't contain dextrose.

Unsweetened Cocoa Powder

Unsweetened cocoa powder will act like self rising flour, while also adding texture and sweetness. That means that you won't have to use as much sweetener. It will also give more depth the recipe.

Chia Seeds

Chia seeds are great to sprinkle on your low carb baking. They soak up liquids, proving fiber and giving your baking the benefit of omega-3 fatty acids. You can even buy it as chia flour. If you choose to use the flour, you'll only have to use half the amount called for in the recipe.

Flax Meal

Flax meal, which consists of ground flax seeds, can be used as a flour substitute. Even though it has a higher fat content than the other four substitutes mentioned above, the fats are of the healthy onega-3 variety. In addition, flax meal is a fantastic source of fiber, meaning that it will fill you up faster.

Become a Label Reader

Getting to grips with the nutritional information on the product label of the food you're eating is going to be essential for you. Carbohydrates are packed into the most unlikely of products, often taking the form of corn syrup, corn starch, and other additives that have zero nutritional value.

Sugar is nearly always added to cured meats, such as sausage, ham, bacon and hot dogs. Eat fresh meats as much as possible. When you do buy cured meats, check the amount of added sugar, as it can vary from 1 gram to 6 grams per serving. If there is no label to read, such as at the deli counter, ask questions.

When a food is labeled as low carb, you may think that you don't have to read the label. In fact, the opposite is true. There are thousands of products flooding into the market in order to cash in on the low carb craze. They may state that they only carry 2 grams of carbohydrate, but when you check the label you come across such ingredients, buried down the list, as corn starch, maltodextrin or sucanat. Be vigilant.

Let's break what you need to look for on the nutritional panel of a label, down using an example so you can extract the information you need. Basically there are 4 major things to focus on to read nutrition labels. They are:

- ✓ Calories
- ✓ Serving Size, (usually at the top of the label)
- ✓ Total Carbohydrate, (usually around the middle of the label and measured in grams)
- ✓ Total Dietary Fiber (just below the total carbs and also measured in grams.

When you subtract the dietary fiber from the total carbs you will get the net carbs per that serving size.

Nutrition Facts

Serving Size 100 g

Amount Per Serving

Calories 250   Calories from fat 10

% Daily Value*

Total Fat 4%	4%
Saturated Fat 1.5%	4%
Trans Fat	
Cholesterol 50mg	28%
Sodium 150mg	15%
Total Carbohydrate 10g	3%
Dietary Fiber 5g	
Sugars 3g	
Protein 16%	

Vitamin A 1%	·	**Vitamin C** 3%	
Calcium 2%	·	Iron 2%	

*Percent Daily Values are based on a 2,000 calorie diet. Your daily values may be higher or lower depending on your calorie needs.

Forty Four Ways to Say Sugar

When checking labels look out for the following sugar laden ingredients:

➢ Agave nectar

- Agave syrup
- Barley malt
- Beet sugar
- Brown rice syrup
- Brown sugar
- Buttered syrup
- Cane sugar
- Cane juice crystals
- Carob syrup
- Confectioner's sugar
- Corn syrup
- Corn sugar
- Corn sweetener
- Corn syrup solids
- Date sugar
- Dextran
- Dextrose
- Diatase
- Diastatic malt
- Evaporated cane juice
- Fructose

- Fruit juice
- Fruit juice concentrate
- Glucose
- Glucose solids
- Golden sugar
- Golden syrup
- Grape sugar
- Grape juice concentrate
- High fructose corn syrup
- Invert sugar
- Lactose
- Malt
- Maltodextrin
- Maltose
- Maple syrup
- Molasses
- Raw sugar
- Refiner's syrup
- Sorghum syrup
- Sucanat
- Turbinado sugar

➤ Yellow sugar

Using the Scale

You can pick up a good set of digital scales for about $20. It will allow you to measure in either grams or ounces.

To measure a food item, set the scale to grams, then place your plate on the scale. Then zero the scale so that the weight of the plate in not added to the weight of the food. Now place your food on the plate. Keep adding food until you hit the serving weight on the food label.

Let's say that you are having a serving of almond flakes, which contains 14 grams of carbs in a 40 gram serving. However, you only want to be eating 5 grams of carbs at this meal. You will need to work out what size serving will provide you with 5 grams of carbs.

You can use a simple calculation to do this . . .

40 divided by 14 = 2.86

5 x 2.86 = 14.3

So, to get your 5 grams of carbs, you will put 14.3 grams of almond flakes on the scale.

Fruits and Vegetable Carbohydrate List

Food	Cal.	Total Carbs	Fiber	Net Carbs	Serving
Asparagus	20	3.7	1.7	2.0	½ cup
Avocado	167	8.7	7.0	1.7	3.5 oz.
Broccoli	27	5.6	2.6	3.0	½ cup
Baby Carrots	32	8.2	2.9	5.3	3.5 oz.
Cauliflower	34	7.0	1.8	2.9	1 cup
Celery	9	1.6	0.67	0.39	2 oz.
Cucumber	4	1.0	0.9	0.18	1 oz.
Garlic	4	1.0	0.9	2.0	1 clove
Green Beans	22	4.9	2.9	1.2	½ cup
Mushrooms	6	0.9	0.61	0.87	1 oz.
Onion, white	16	7.5	6.0	0.88	½ cup
Pepper, Sweet	6	1.3	0.8	0.2	1 oz.
Pickles, Dill	7	1.5	1.0	0.3	1 oz.
Romaine Lettuce	5	0.9	0.3	0.3	1 oz.
Butter head Lettuce	4	0.7	0.4	0.4	1 oz.
Shallots	20	4.7	4.0	0.7	1 oz.
Snow Peas	34	5.6	3.4	2.6	½ cup
Spinach	33	5.0	2.0	4.0	5 oz.
Squash, Butternut	82	6.8	15	1.8	1 cup cubes
Tomato	5	1.0	0.7	0.2	1 oz.

Chapter 4: Seven Day Meal Plan

The key to a successful ketogenic meal plan is preparation. By pre-cooking your meals, you are giving yourself a huge advantage. The biggest challenge to any new eating regime comes when you're under time pressure, you're fatigued and starving. That usually happens mid-week around dinner time. Being able to simply pull a pre-made keto meal from the freezer and pop it into the microwave could be a life-saver.

We suggest **preparing** your meals on a Sunday. Purchase individual sized Tupperware containers to allow you to apportion out your food. You'll find all of the recipes used in this meal plan in the Recipes section to follow.

Your Seven-Day Meal Plan

Day 1 –Seven Day Meal Plan

1) *Breakfast*

Avocado Baked Eggs

- ➢ Calories: 372
- ➢ Fats: 32g
- ➢ Net Carbs: 6g
- ➢ Protein: 16g

2) *Lunch*

Quesadilla with Creamy Mushroom Dip

- ➢ Calories: 404
- ➢ Fats: 43g
- ➢ Net Carbs: 2.4g
- ➢ Protein: 21g

3) *Dinner*

Pickled Salmon

- ➢ Calories: 170
- ➢ Fats: 4g
- ➢ Net Carbs: 7g
- ➢ Protein: 23g

Day 2 –Seven Day Meal Plan

1) *Breakfast*

Maple Flavored Pork Bake

- ➢ Calories: 405
- ➢ Fats: 37g
- ➢ Net Carbs: 17g

➤ Protein: 1.9g

2) *Lunch*

Veal Picata
➤ Calories: 325
➤ Fats: 20g
➤ Net Carbs: 1g
➤ Protein: 32g

3) *Dinner*

Bacon Chili Burgers
➤ Calories: 485
➤ Fats: 38g
➤ Net Carbs: 2g
➤ Protein: 31g

Day 3 –Seven Day Meal Plan

1) *Breakfast*

Avocado Tuna Melt Bites
➤ Calories: 352
➤ Fats: 36g
➤ Net Carbs: 5.5g
➤ Protein: 25g

2) *Lunch*

Curried Chicken Salad
- ➢ Calories: 318
- ➢ Fats: 24g
- ➢ Net Carbs: 3g
- ➢ Protein: 22g

3) *Dinner*

Orange Tequila Steak
- ➢ Calories: 560
- ➢ Fats: 46g
- ➢ Net Carbs: 5g
- ➢ Protein: 26g

Day 4 –Seven Day Meal Plan

1) *Breakfast*

Avocado Baked Eggs
- ➢ Calories: 372
- ➢ Fats: 32g
- ➢ Net Carbs: 6g
- ➢ Protein: 16g

2) *Lunch*

Tandoori Chicken
- ➢ Calories: 503
- ➢ Fats: 30g
- ➢ Net Carbs: 4g

> ➤ Protein: 52g

3) *Dinner*

Smoky Marinated Steak
> ➤ Calories: 276
> ➤ Fats: 20g
> ➤ Net Carbs: 1g
> ➤ Protein: 23g

Day 5 –Seven Day Meal Plan

1) *Breakfast*

Breakfast Casserole
> ➤ Calories: 276
> ➤ Fats: 20g
> ➤ Net Carbs: 1g
> ➤ Protein: 23g

2) *Lunch*

Quesadilla with Creamy Mushroom Dip
> ➤ Calories: 404
> ➤ Fats: 43g
> ➤ Net Carbs: 2.4g
> ➤ Protein: 21g

3) *Dinner*

Pickled Salmon
  - ➤ Calories: 170
  - ➤ Fats: 4g
  - ➤ Net Carbs: 7g
  - ➤ Protein: 23g

Day 6 – Seven Day Meal Plan

1) *Breakfast*

Maple Flavored Pork Bake
  - ➤ Calories: 405
  - ➤ Fats: 37g
  - ➤ Net Carbs: 17g
  - ➤ Protein: 1.9g

2) *Lunch*

Veal Picata
  - ➤ Calories: 325
  - ➤ Fats: 20g
  - ➤ Net Carbs: 1g
  - ➤ Protein: 32g

3) *Dinner*

Bacon Chili Burgers
  - ➤ Calories: 485

- ➢ Fats: 38g
- ➢ Net Carbs: 2g
- ➢ Protein: 31g

Day 7 –Seven Day Meal Plan

1) Breakfast

Avocado Tuna Melt Bites
- ➢ Calories: 372
- ➢ Fats: 32g
- ➢ Net Carbs: 6g
- ➢ Protein: 16g

2) Lunch

Curried Chicken Salad
- ➢ Calories: 318
- ➢ Fats: 24g
- ➢ Net Carbs: 3g
- ➢ Protein: 22g

3) Dinner

Orange Tequila Steak
- ➢ Calories: 560
- ➢ Fats: 46g
- ➢ Net Carbs: 5g
- ➢ Protein: 26g

Chapter 5: The Recipes

Breakfast

Creamy Parmesan Eggs

Prep Time: 2 minutes
Cooking Time: 16 minutes
Serves: 1

Ingredients:
- ✓ 2 large eggs
- ✓ ¾ tablespoon heavy cream
- ✓ 1/8 tablespoon Parmesan cheese
- ✓ ½ teaspoon butter

Steps:
- ✓ Preheat the oven to 325°F. Grease a ramekin or coat it with non-stick cooking spray.
1) Crack the eggs into the ramekin.
2) Float 11/2 tablespoons of heavy cream on top of the eggs.
3) Scatter the Parmesan cheese on top. Dab the butter on top of this.
4) Place the ramekin in the oven and bake for 16 minutes.
5) Serve your eggs hot.

Nutritional Breakdown: 248 calories, 20 grams' fat, 14 grams protein, 2 grams total carbs, 0 grams dietary fiber.

Note: A ramekin is a small glazed bowel used for backing and serving food. It usually is made from glass or earthenware. Get your best value ramekin set here: http://amzn.to/1TpPE9m

Avocado Baked Eggs

Prep Time: 3 minutes
Cooking Time: 12 minutes
Serves: 1

Ingredients:

- ✓ 1 slice of bacon
- ✓ ½ an avocado, not too squishy, pip removed
- ✓ ¼ teaspoon Creole seasoning
- ✓ 1 large egg
- ✓ 1 oz. Monterey Jack cheese, shredded or sliced

Steps:
1) Preheat the oven to 400°F.

1) Fry the bacon until it is crisp.
2) Scoop out a little flesh from the cavity of the avocado to allow it to fit an egg.
3) Take a sharp knife and score the flesh of the avocado in a crisscross pattern so that you create ½ inch squares.
4) Grease a ramekin or coat it with non-stick cooking spray.
5) Place the avocado half in the ramekin.
6) Spoon some bacon grease onto the avocado, allowing it to get into the scoring. Sprinkle on the Creole seasoning.
7) Break the egg into the avocado half.
8) Place the ramekin in the oven and cook for 12 minutes. After 10 minutes, pull out and sprinkle with cheese.
9) Garnish with the bacon and serve.

Nutritional Breakdown: 372 calories, 32 grams fat, 16 grams protein, 9 grams total carbs, 3 grams dietary fiber.

Creamy Asparagus Frittata

Prep Time: 2 minutes
Cooking Time: 16 minutes
Serves: 1

Ingredients:

- ✓ ½ tablespoon butter
- ✓ 1/8 small onion
- ✓ 1/8-pound asparagus
- ✓ 1 large egg
- ✓ ¼ cup shredded Swiss cheese
- ✓ ¼ cup grated Parmesan cheese
- ✓ 1/8 cup of dry white wine
- ✓ 1/8 cup of heavy cream
- ✓ 1/8 teaspoon of dried thyme
- ✓ 1/8 teaspoon salt

Steps:
1) Coat a skillet with cooking spray and place it over a medium-low heat. Melt the butter and start sautéing the onion.
2) Snap the ends off the asparagus and cut into ½ inch lengths.
3) Whisk all the other ingredients in a bowl.
4) When the onion is soft, add the asparagus to the skillet and sauté it until it turns bright green (about 1 minute).
5) Add the eggs and stir so the onion and egg are evenly distributed.
6) Reduce to a low heat, cover and cook for 15 minutes.
7) Turn on the broiler and slide the skillet into the oven so that it is about 6 inches

from the heat. Broil until the top becomes golden.

Nutritional Breakdown: 238 calories, 18 grams fat, 13 grams protein, 4 grams total carbs, 1 grams dietary fiber.

Avocado Tuna Melts

Prep Time: 4 minutes
Cooking Time: 7 minutes
Serves: 1

Ingredients:

- ✓ 1 can drained tuna
- ✓ ¼ cup of mayonnaise
- ✓ 1 small avocado, cubed
- ✓ ¼ cup Parmesan cheese
- ✓ ½ tablespoon garlic powder
- ✓ ¼ tablespoon onion powder
- ✓ salt and pepper to taste
- ✓ ¼ cup coconut oil for frying
- ✓ I cup almond flour

Steps:
1) Drain the tuna and place it into a large bowl.

2) Add in mayonnaise, Parmesan cheese and spices and mix well.
3) Add the avocado cubes into the mixture, without squashing them.
4) Form the mixture into balls and roll in almond flour until completely covered.
5) Heat the coconut oil in a pan and cook the tuna balls until they are crisp all over. Serve immediately.

Nutritional Breakdown: 352 calories, 36 grams fat, 25 grams protein, 14 grams total carbs, 7.5 grams dietary fiber.

Maple Flavored Pork Bake

Prep Time: 2 minutes
Cooking Time: 16 minutes
Serves: 1

Ingredients:

- ✓ 1.5 oz. 40% heavy cream, whipped
- ✓ 3 drops of vanilla flavoring
- ✓ 6 oz. ground pork, cooked
- ✓ ½ oz. macadamia nuts, crushed
- ✓ 0.4 oz. butter
- ✓ 1 oz. cheddar cheese
- ✓ pinch of calorie free sweetener

✓ 3 drops maple flavoring

Steps:
1) Mix the whipped cream with the vanilla flavour and half of the sweetener.
2) Freeze for 15 minutes.
3) Pre-heat the oven to 350 degrees F. In an oven safe dish, mix the pork, macadamia nuts, butter, cheese, remaining sweetener, and maple flavor. Bake for 15 minutes.
4) Serve with the frozen whipped cream on top as ice cream.

Nutritional Breakdown: 405 calories, 37 grams fat, 17 grams protein, 6 grams total carbs, 4.1 grams dietary fiber.

Pork Bagel

Prep Time: 7 minutes
Cooking Time: 40 minutes
Serves: 1

Ingredients:
✓ ¾ onion minced
✓ ¼lb. organic ground lean pork
✓ ½ tablespoon butter
✓ ½ cup sugar free tomato sauce

✓ 1 large egg
✓ ½ teaspoon sea salt
✓ ½ teaspoon paprika
✓ ¼ teaspoon freshly ground paprika

Steps:

1) Pre-heat the oven to 400 degrees F. Line a baking dish with parchment paper.
2) Place a non-stick skillet over a medium flame and melt the butter.
3) Add the onions, cooking until they are translucent. Take off the heat and put aside to cool.
4) In a bowl, mix the ground pork, tomato sauce, eggs, salt, pepper, paprika and onions.
5) Divide the mixture into 3 balls. Press each ball in the middle and flatten it out to look like a bagel.
6) Place the bagels in the cooking dish and bake for 40 minutes, or until they are firm.
7) Serve warm.

Nutritional Breakdown: 239 calories, 36 grams fat, 22 grams protein, 7 grams total carbs, 2.1 grams dietary fiber.

Note: A digital scale will help you stay honest on your keto weight loss plan. Measuring by weight will help your recipe true. Check out

the best price on digital kitchen scales here:
http://amzn.to/1TIhbPo

Yogurt and Chia Seed Parfait

Prep Time: 7 minutes
Cooking Time: 0 minutes
Serves: 1

Ingredients:

- ✓ 1 cup full fat yogurt
- ✓ 2 tablespoons chia seeds
- ✓ 1/4 teaspoon cinnamon
- ✓ ¼ cup unsweetened almond milk
- ✓ 2 Tablespoons sliced almonds

Steps:

1) Combine the almond milk, chia seeds and yogurt in a bowl.
2) Pour one layer of the mixture into a glass.
3) Add the almonds and cinnamon.
4) Repeat this process until you have 3 layers.
5) Refrigerate the glass for 12 minutes to thicken the parfait. Serve chilled.

Nutritional Breakdown: 212 calories, 35 grams fat, 13 grams protein, 8 grams total carbs, 3.2 grams dietary fiber.

Breakfast Casserole

Prep Time: 6 minutes
Cooking Time: 25 minutes
Serves: 1

Ingredients:

- ✓ 2 large eggs
- ✓ ¼ lb. sausage
- ✓ ½ cup of grated cheddar cheese
- ✓ ½ cup heavy cream
- ✓ ¼ head cauliflower
- ✓ ¼ teaspoon dry mustard
- ✓ ¼ teaspoon sea salt

Steps:
1) Preheat the oven to 350°F. Grease a casserole dish or coat it with non-stick cooking spray.
2) Place a non-stick skillet over a medium-high flame and cook the sausage until browned and crumbled.
3) Scrape the sausage into a bowl, then stir in the chopped cauliflower, heavy cream,

cheese, salt and mustard. Set aside to cool.

4) Whisk the eggs in a separate bowl, then stir into the sausage mixture.
5) Pour the mixture into the casserole dish. Bake for 25 minutes.
6) Set on a wire rack to cool slightly, then serve.

Nutritional Breakdown: 311 calories, 32 grams fat, 18 grams protein, 8.6 grams total carbs, 2.8 grams dietary fiber.

Cauliflower Waffles

Prep Time: 2 minutes
Cooking Time: 16 minutes
Serves: 1

Ingredients:

- ✓ 2 eggs
- ✓ ¼ cup mozzarella cheese
- ✓ ¾ cup coarsely ground cauliflower
- ✓ 1 ½ teaspoons chopped, fresh chives
- ✓ ¼ teaspoon garlic powder
- ✓ ¼ teaspoon onion powder
- ✓ red pepper flakes
- ✓ sea salt

✓ freshly ground black pepper

Steps:
1) Place the cauliflower and cheese in a food processor. Pulse until thoroughly mixed.
2) Add eggs, chives, garlic and onion powder, along with a dash of each of red pepper flakes, salt and black pepper. Process well.
3) Pour the mixture into the waffle maker and cook according to manufacturer's instructions.
4) Place the waffles on a plate and serve with yogurt, cream cheese, and/or crumbled bacon. Sere immediately.

Nutritional Breakdown: 198 calories, 720 grams fat, 16 grams protein, 6 grams total fat, 2.1 grams dietary fiber.

Note: A food processor is an essential tool in the keto kitchen. You'll want a processor that comes with special blades and disc attachments that allow it to mince, grate, shred. Chop, knead, blend puree and liquefy. You'll also want a unit that has a cover over the work bowl with a feeder tube that allows you to feed ingredients in while it is operating.

Find the best deal on food processors here:
http://amzn.to/1R9GuYB

Chic-Can Pie

Prep Time: 10 minutes
Cooking Time: 20 minutes
Serves: 1

Ingredients:

- ✓ ⅛ cup pecan nuts
- ✓ ½ teaspoon lard
- ✓ ¼ small onion, diced
- ✓ 1 small handful of shredded cheese
- ✓ Savory pastry (you can find a good selection of pre-made savory pastry at your local grocery store)
- ✓ ¼ cup shredded chicken
- ✓ 1 egg
- ✓ 2 Tablespoons cream
- ✓ Pinch of Paprika (to taste)
- ✓ Salt and pepper (to taste)

Steps:
1) Preheat your oven to 325°F.
2) Lay the nuts in a roasting dish and place them in the oven for five minutes to lightly roast.
3) Melt the lard in a skillet and sauté the onion until they are soft and translucent.

4) Place the pastry in a single serve pie dish or in a deep dish muffin tin.
5) Start assembling the pie - start with a layer of cheese, then add the chicken, top with the pecans.
6) Combine the wet ingredients, the paprika and the salt and pepper. Whisk together and pour over the pie filling.
7) Bake for 20 minutes.

Nutritional Breakdown: 577 calories; 46g fat; 32g protein; 13g carbohydrate; 2g dietary fiber

Moorish Mushroom Omelet

Prep Time: 10 minutes
Cooking Time: 20 minutes
Serves: 1

Ingredients:

- ✓ 1 Tablespoon finely chopped onion
- ✓ 1 small handful sliced mushrooms
- ✓ ·2 Tablespoons butter
- ✓ 2 large eggs
- ✓ 1 small handful shredded cheese (I recommend Swiss)
- ✓ Pinch of nutmeg
- ✓ Salt and Pepper (to taste)

Steps:
1) Melt half of the butter in a skillet and sauté the mushroom and onions until they are soft. Transfer them onto a plate and reserve for later in the recipe.
2) Place the skillet back on the heat and melt the second half of the butter.
3) Whisk the eggs, nutmeg, salt and pepper in a bowl and then transfer to the hot skillet.
4) Move the skillet so the egg mixture covers the entire bottom of the skillet and cook until the egg is almost done.
5) When the egg is almost set, add the cheese, mushrooms on top of the egg mix, folding the omelet over.
6) Enjoy immediately.

Nutritional Breakdown: 513 calories; 44g fat; 25g protein; 6g carbohydrate; 1g dietary fiber

Butter Mushroom and Swiss Omelet

Prep Time: 2 minutes
Cooking Time: 6 minutes
Serves: 1

Ingredients:

- ✓ 1/2 tablespoon (10 g) minced onion
- ✓ 1 ounces (55 g) mushrooms, sliced
- ✓ 1 tablespoon (28 g) butter, divided
- ✓ Pinch of ground nutmeg
- ✓ 1 large egg
- ✓ 3/4 oz. Swiss cheese, sliced or shredded

Steps:
1) Mince the onion and slice the mushrooms.
2) Melt the butter over medium heat in a skillet.
3) Sauté the onion and mushrooms with the nutmeg until they are soft. Remove to a plate.
4) Scramble the eggs. Pour the eggs into the skillet over a high heat. Add the sautéed ingredients and top with Swiss cheese.

Nutritional Breakdown: 513 calories; 44g fat; 25g protein; 6g carbohydrate; 1g dietary fiber

Coconut Cornflakes

Prep Time: 5 minutes
Cooking Time: 30 minutes
Serves: 1

Ingredients:

- ✓ 1 cups flaked coconut
- ✓ 1/4 teaspoon salt
- ✓ 1/8 teaspoon liquid Stevia
- ✓ 1/2 teaspoon vanilla extract
- ✓ 1/8 cup water
- ✓ 1/8 cup powdered Swerve

Steps:
1) Preheat oven to 325 degrees F. Line a shallow baking pan with aluminum foil.
2) Put the coconut flakes in a large bowl.
3) Stir the salt, Stevia and vanilla extract into the water until the salt is dissolved.
4) Sprinkle the seasoned water over the coconut, a tablespoon at a time. Be sure to mix thoroughly.
5) Add the swerve to evenly coat the coconut.
6) Spread the coconut in an even layer on the baking pan.
7) Bake for 15 minutes. Stir well, spread out evenly and bake for a further 15 minutes. Stir every 5 minutes.
8) Remove to cool and then serve.

Nutritional Breakdown: 143 calories; 13g fat; 1g protein; 6g carbohydrate; 4g dietary fiber

Flax and Coconut Pancakes

Prep Time: 30 minutes
Cooking Time: 2 minutes
Serves: 1

Ingredients:

- ✓ 1/4 cup flaxseed meal
- ✓ 1/4 cup shredded coconut
- ✓ 1/4 teaspoon baking soda
- ✓ 1/4 teaspoon salt
- ✓ 1/4 cup sour cream or Coconut Sour Cream
- ✓ 1 large egg
- ✓ 1/8 teaspoon liquid stevia

Steps:
1) Mix all the ingredients together in a bowl.
2) Pour into a skillet on a medium heat and cook for 1 minute on either side.
3) Serve with a side of bacon.

Nutritional Breakdown: 141 calories; 11g fat; 6g protein; 6g carbohydrate; 5g dietary fiber

Lunch

Quesadilla with Creamy Mushroom Dip

Prep Time: 3 minutes
Cooking Time: 5 minutes
Serves: 1

Ingredients:

- ✓ 1/8 cup heavy duty cream
- ✓ 1 Tablespoon mayonnaise
- ✓ 1 Teaspoon olive oil
- ✓ 1 avocado
- ✓ Dollop of butter
- ✓ 2 egg whites
- ✓ 1/8 cup almond flour
- ✓ Grated cheese to garnish

Steps:
1) Combine the cream, olive oil, avocado and mayonnaise in a mixing bowl. Mash together until smooth.
2) In another bowl, mix the egg whites and almond flour.
3) Melt the butter in a small non-stick fry-pan on medium heat.
4) Pour the egg whites into the pan in a thin layer.

5) When the egg mixture is opaque, flip and cook the other side.
6) Remove the heat and add the cheese, sprinkling it on top.
7) Fold in half to melt the cheese.
8) Remove eggs from the pan and slice into wedges. Serve with avocado dip.

Nutritional Breakdown: 404 calories; 43g fat; 21g protein; 7.1g carbohydrate; 4.6g dietary fiber

Chilled Avocado Soup

Prep Time: 3 minutes
Cooking Time: 15 minutes
Serves: 1

Ingredients:

- ½ tablespoon canola oil
- 1/8 cup chopped yellow onion
- 1/4 clove minced garlic
- ½ cup chicken broth
- ¼ cup milk
- ½ ripe avocado, peeled, pitted and cubed
- ¼ teaspoon fresh lime juice
- ½ teaspoon course salt

- ✓ 1/4 teaspoon freshly ground pepper
- ✓ ¼ teaspoon Tabasco sauce
- ✓ ¼ teaspoon chopped fresh chives

Steps:

1) Heat a saucepan for 2 minutes.
2) Add oil and swirl to coat the pan evenly.
3) Add onion and garlic, sautéing for 2 minutes.
4) Add chicken broth and milk, bringing the mixture to the boil.
5) Cover, reduce the heat and allow the mixture to simmer for 10 minutes.
6) Turn off the heat and put aside the pan for 10 minutes to cool.
7) Place the avocado, lime juice, salt, pepper and Tabasco sauce in a food processor and mix until well chopped. Add the chicken broth mixture and blend until smooth.
8) Transfer your soup to a large bowl. Serve immediately.

Nutritional Breakdown: 271 calories; 24g fat; 5g protein; 12g carbohydrate; 5g dietary fiber, sodium 791 mg

Curried Chicken Salad

Prep Time: 6 minutes
Cooking Time: 30 minutes
Serves: 1

Ingredients:

- ✓ 1/4 clove garlic
- ✓ ¼ teaspoon chopped fresh ginger
- ✓ ½ teaspoon fresh lemon juice
- ✓ 1/4 teaspoon curry powder
- ✓ ¼ teaspoon Dijon mustard
- ✓ ¼ teaspoon coarse salt
- ✓ ¼ teaspoon freshly ground pepper
- ✓ ¼ cup canola oil
- ✓ 1 cup cooked and cubed chicken
- ✓ ½ cup broccoli florets, blanched for 1 minute
- ✓ ½ cup sliced celery
- ✓ ¼ cup salted cashews
- ✓ 1 cup pre-washed spinach
- ✓ chives, to garnish

Steps:

1) To make the curry vinaigrette, chop up the garlic and ginger in a food processor. Add the lemon juice, curry, mustard and salt and pepper and blend. Pour the canola oil and process until smooth. Put this mixture in a container and cool in the fridge for an hour.

2) Combine the chicken, broccoli, celery and cashews in a large bowl. Add the curry vinaigrette and toss until well blended.

3) To serve, make a bed of the spinach on a dinner plate. Spoon the salad in the middle of the spinach. Garnish with long strands of chives.

Nutritional Breakdown: 318 calories; 24g fat;22g protein; 5g carbohydrate; 2g dietary fiber, sodium 213 mg

Note: A salad spinner is the fastest way to dry salad greens and herbs. Some salad spinners even combine washing and drying functions. Check out a great salad spinner deal here: **http://amzn.to/1WDwks2**

Pork Tenderloin

Prep Time: 5 minutes (plus overnight refrigeration)
Cooking Time: 50 minutes
Serves: 1

Ingredients:
- ✓ 1/4 tablespoon canola oil
- ✓ ¼ tablespoon hot pepper sauce
- ✓ ¼ tablespoon artificial sweetener

- ✓ ¼ tablespoon soy sauce
- ✓ ¼ tablespoon minced fresh ginger
- ✓ ½ teaspoon chopped green onion
- ✓ ½ teaspoon Asian sesame oil
- ✓ ¼ clove minced garlic
- ✓ ½ pound pork tenderloin

Steps:
1. To make the marinade combine all of the ingredients apart from the pork in a large plastic bag and mix well. Add the pork tenderloin and turn to fully coat it. Seal the bag and refrigerate overnight.
2. Preheat oven to 325 degrees F. Lightly coat a shallow pan with a non-stick vegetable spray.
3. Remove the pork tenderloin from the marinade, reserving the marinade. Place the pork in the pan. Bake for 50 minutes. Every 15 minutes, apply a baste of the marinade.
4. Cool for 10 minutes and then carve into thin slices.

Nutritional Breakdown: 257 calories; 11g fat;36g protein; 1g carbohydrate; 0g dietary fiber, sodium 330 mg

Greek Chicken

Prep Time: 5 minutes (plus overnight refrigeration)
Cooking Time: 50 minutes
Serves: 1

Ingredients:
- ✓ ½ tablespoon Greek dried oregano leaves
- ✓ ¼ tablespoon ground Oregano
- ✓ ½ teaspoon salt
- ✓ ½ teaspoon freshly ground pepper
- ✓ ¼ teaspoon thyme leaves
- ✓ ¼ clove minced garlic
- ✓ ¼ chicken, all visible fat removed

Steps:
1) Make the Greek rub by combining all the ingredients apart from the chicken in a small bowl and mixing well.
2) Press the rub on both sides of the chicken.
3) Place the chicken in a plastic bag and cool in the fridge overnight.
4) Place the chicken on a grill coated with non-stick vegetable spray. Cover the grill and cook, turning every 5 minutes, for 30-40 minutes.
5) Serve immediately.

Nutritional Breakdown:471 calories; 28g fat;50g protein; 3g carbohydrate; 0g dietary fiber, sodium 1092 mg

Lemon and Tarragon Marinated Salmon

Prep Time: 15 minutes
Cooking Time: 30 minutes
Serves: 1

Ingredients:

- ✓ 1/8 cup fresh lemon juice
- ✓ ¼ tablespoon extra virgin olive oil
- ✓ ¼ tablespoon fresh tarragon
- ✓ 1/8 teaspoon coarse salt
- ✓ 1/8 teaspoon freshly ground pepper
- ✓ 1 salmon fillet (6 oz.)
- ✓ Thinly sliced lemon to garnish

Steps:
1) To make the marinade, combine all ingredients except the salmon in a dish, mixing well.
2) Add the salmon filet, and coat it liberally. Cover and refrigerate for 30 minutes.
3) Remove the fillet from the marinade, and place on a grill coated with a non-

stick vegetable spray over a medium heat. Grill for 10 minutes.
4) Garnish with a slice of lemon

Nutritional Breakdown: 279 calories; 14g fat;34g protein; 2g carbohydrate; 0g dietary fiber, sodium 196 mg

Tandoori Chicken

Prep Time: 5 minutes (plus refrigeration overnight)
Cooking Time: 35 minutes
Serves: 1

Ingredients:
- ¼ cup plain yogurt
- ½ tablespoon fresh lime juice
- ¼ piece of fresh ginger, peeled and minced
- ¼ garlic, minced
- ¼ teaspoon chili powder
- ¼ teaspoon coarse salt
- 1/8 teaspoon ground cumin
- 1/8 teaspoon ground turmeric
- ¼ tablespoon tandoori paste
- ¼ chicken, with all visible fat removed

Steps:

1) To make the marinade put all the ingredients excluding the chicken in a large re-sealable bag. Shake well.
2) Add the chicken and coat liberally. Refrigerate overnight.
3) Remove the chicken from the marinade and place on a grill coated with a non-stick vegetable spray over medium heat. Grill for 35 minutes. Baste a couple of times with the marinade.
4) Serve immediately.

Nutritional Breakdown: 503 calories; 30g fat;52g protein; 4g carbohydrate; 0g dietary fiber, sodium 164 mg

Asian Green Bean Stir Fry

Prep Time: 5 minutes
Cooking Time: 10 minutes
Serves: 1

Ingredients:

- ✓ 11/2 tablespoons chicken broth
- ✓ ½ tablespoon soy sauce
- ✓ ½ tablespoon Asian sesame sauce
- ✓ ¼ pound green deans, trimmed
- ✓ ¼ clove garlic, minced

- ✓ ¼ tablespoon minced fresh finger
- ✓ ¼ tablespoon toasted sesame seeds

Steps:

1) Combine the chicken broth and soy sauce in a bowl and mix vigorously. Set aside.
2) Heat a skillet for 60 seconds. Add sesame oil, allowing it to coat the bottom of the pan. Add green beans, stir-frying for 5 minutes. Add the chicken stock mixture, garlic and ginger and stir-fry for 1 minute.
3) Cover the skillet, cooking for 2 minutes.
4) Remove the cover and continue cooking until there is no liquid left in the skillet.
5) Sprinkle with sesame seeds.

Nutritional Breakdown: 64 calories; 2g fat;3g protein; 9g carbohydrate; 4g dietary fiber, sodium 617 mg

Cuban Pork Loin Roast

Prep Time: 5 minutes (plus refrigeration overnight)
Cooking Time: 120 minutes
Serves: 1

Ingredients:
- ✓ 8 cup fresh orange juice
- ✓ ¼ tablespoon fresh lime juice
- ✓ 1/8 tablespoon extra virgin olive oil
- ✓ 1/4 clove garlic, minced
- ✓ 1/8 teaspoon ground cumin
- ✓ 1/8 teaspoon dried oregano leaves
- ✓ 1/8 teaspoon coarse salt
- ✓ 1/8 teaspoon freshly ground pepper
- ✓ pork loin boneless roast (1/2 pound)

Steps:
1) Make the orange juice marinade by combining all the ingredients, with the exception of the pork in a re-sealable bag and mixing well.
2) Add the pork roast and coat it liberally. Seal the bag and refrigerate overnight.
3) Pre-heat the oven to 325 degrees F. Place the pork roast in a roasting pan and pour the marinade over top. Bake for 2 hours.
4) Cool for at least 10 minutes before carving into slices.

Nutritional Breakdown: 369 calories; 15g fat;52g protein; 3g carbohydrate; 0g dietary fiber, sodium 133 mg

Note: A meat thermometer is the most accurate measure of when your meats are ready. Simply insert it into the cooked meat to get instant readout of the internal temperature. Check out the best price on meat thermometers here: **http://amzn.to/208iXOc**

New Delhi Turkey Meatloaf

Prep Time: 5 minutes
Cooking Time: 95 minutes
Serves: 1

Ingredients:

- ✓ 1/4 tablespoon extra virgin olive oil
- ✓ 1/4 clove garlic, minced
- ✓ 1/8 teaspoon ground cumin
- ✓ 1/8 cup chopped yellow onion
- ✓ 1/8 teaspoon coarse salt
- ✓ 1/8 teaspoon freshly ground pepper
- ✓ 1/8 teaspoon freshly ground coriander
- ✓ 1/8 teaspoon freshly ground cinnamon
- ✓ 1/8 teaspoon cayenne pepper
- ✓ ½ pound ground turkey
- ✓ ½ egg, lightly beaten
- ✓ 1/8 teaspoon Dijon mustard

Steps:

1) Pre-heat oven to 325-degree F. Lightly coat a 9 x 5-inch loaf pan with non-stick vegetable spray. Set aside.
2) Heat a medium non-stick skillet over medium heat for 2 minutes. Add the olive oil and swirl the pan to coat the bottom evenly.
3) Add onion, garlic, curry, ginger, salt, pepper, coriander, cumin, cinnamon, and cayenne and sauté for 5 minutes. Then remove from heat and cool for 10 minutes.
4) Combine the turkey, onion mixture, egg and mustard in a bowl and mix well. Place in the prepared pan and press down to make it evenly flat.
5) Bake for 85 minutes. Then remove from the oven and drain off as much fat as possible.
6) Cut into slices and serve immediately.

Nutritional Breakdown: 247 calories; 17g fat;22g protein; 2g carbohydrate; 1g dietary fiber, sodium 133 mg

Veal Picata

Prep Time: 5 minutes
Cooking Time: 8 minutes

Serves: 1

Ingredients:

- ✓ 1/4 tablespoon extra virgin olive oil
- ✓ 1 veal scallop (6 oz.)
- ✓ 1/8 teaspoon coarse salt
- ✓ 1/8 teaspoon freshly ground pepper
- ✓ 1/8 teaspoon freshly ground coriander
- ✓ ¼ garlic clove, minced
- ✓ 1/8 cup chicken broth
- ✓ 1/8 cup fresh lemon juice
- ✓ ½ tablespoon capers, rinsed and drained
- ✓ ½ tablespoon butter
- ✓ ½ tablespoon minced fresh parsley
- ✓ thinly sliced lemon for garnish

Steps:

1) Heat a skillet for 60 seconds. Add olive oil and swirl the pan to coat the bottom evenly. Season both sides of the veal with salt and pepper. Place the veal in the skillet and sauté for 2 minutes on each side. Remove to a plate and cover with foil.
2) Add the garlic to the skillet and sauté for 30 seconds. Add chicken broth and cook on high for 2 minutes. Add lemon juice and capers and cook for 1 minute.

3) Remove the skillet from the heat and add the butter. Once butter has melted add the parsley and blend.
4) Garnish with a lemon slice to serve.

Nutritional Breakdown: 325 calories; 20g fat;32g protein; 2g carbohydrate; 1g dietary fiber, sodium 595 mg

<u>Spicy Tofu</u>

Prep Time: 5 minutes
Cooking Time: 25 minutes
Serves: 1

Ingredients:
- ✓ 1/4 package extra firm tofu (4 oz.)
- ✓ 1/2 tablespoon Asian sesame oil
- ✓ 1/2 tablespoon soy sauce
- ✓ 1/2 teaspoon red wine vinegar
- ✓ 1 clove garlic, minced
- ✓ 1/4 teaspoon ground coriander
- ✓ 1/4 teaspoon ground turmeric
- ✓ 1/4 teaspoon dried basil
- ✓ 1/4 teaspoon dried marjoram leaves
- ✓ 1/4 teaspoon dried red pepper flakes
- ✓ ¼ teaspoon coarse salt
- ✓ ¼ teaspoon freshly ground pepper

Steps:

1) Place the tofu on a double thickness of paper towels and blot dry.
2) Cut the tofu in half and put aside.
3) To make the marinade, combine the remainder of the ingredients in a dish and mix well. Add the tofu and turn to coat all over. Cover and put in the fridge to cool overnight.
4) Pre-heat oven to 375 degrees F. Lightly coat a rimmed baking sheet with non-stick vegetable spray.
5) Remove the tofu from the marinade, place on the baling sheet and bake for 25 minutes. Serve immediately.

Nutritional Breakdown: 99 calories; 6g fat;9g protein; 3g carbohydrate; 1g dietary fiber, sodium 447 mg

Asparagus with Orange Sauce

Prep Time: 2 minutes
Cooking Time: 7 minutes
Serves: 1

Ingredients:

- ✓ 1/8 cup butter
- ✓ 1/8 cup fresh orange juice

✓ 1/2 tablespoon finely grated orange rind
✓ 1/2-pound fresh asparagus spears tough ends removed

Steps:

1) To make the orange sauce, combine the butter, orange juice and orange rind in a small saucepan over a medium heat. Cook for 4-5 minutes.
2) Bring salted water to a rolling boil in a large skillet. Add asparagus and blanch for 1-2 minutes until crisp.
3) Transfer asparagus to a colander, rinsing thoroughly in cold water. Dry with a paper towel.
4) Drizzle orange juice over asparagus to serve.

Nutritional Breakdown: 136 calories; 12g fat;3g protein; 7g carbohydrate; 3g dietary fiber, sodium 4 mg

Green Beans with Almonds

Prep Time: 2 minutes
Cooking Time: 7 minutes
Serves: 1

Ingredients:

- ✓ ¼ pound green beans, trimmed
- ✓ 1 tablespoon butter
- ✓ 1/8 cup sliced almonds
- ✓ 1/8 teaspoon coarse salt
- ✓ 1/8 teaspoon freshly ground pepper

Steps:

1) Bring salted water to a rolling boil in a large saucepan over high heat.
2) Add green beans and cook for 6 minutes, until crisp. Transfer green beans to a colander and rinse with cold water. Dry with a paper towel.
3) Melt butter in a large skillet over medium heat. Add almonds, salt and pepper and sauté for 2 minutes, stirring frequently.
4) Add green beans and sauté for 2 minutes, stirring frequently.

Nutritional Breakdown: 183 calories; 15g fat;5g protein; 10g carbohydrate; 5g dietary fiber, sodium 126 mg

Dinner

Pickled Salmon

Prep Time: 5 minutes (plus refrigeration overnight)
Cooking Time: 20 minutes
Serves: 1

Ingredients:

- ✓ 1/2-pound salmon steaks or skinned fillets
- ✓ 1 teaspoon salt
- ✓ 1 cup water
- ✓ 1/4 cup white vinegar
- ✓ 1/4 cup Splenda
- ✓ 1/4 bay leaf
- ✓ 1-inch piece cinnamon stick
- ✓ 1/4 slice fresh ginger crushed
- ✓ 1/4 lemon sliced
- ✓ 1/2 medium onion, thinly sliced

Steps:
1) Rub the fish with the salt and then refrigerate for one hour.
2) Combine the water, Splenda, vinegar, bay leaf, cinnamon stick, ginger and lemon in a saucepan. Bring the mixture to the boil, lower the heat and allow to simmer for 5 minutes.

3) Add the fish and simmer uncovered for another 7 minutes.
4) Place onion slices on a casserole dish and with the fish on top and cover with the hot vinegar mixture. Cover and refrigerate overnight.

Nutritional Breakdown: 170 calories; 4g fat;23g protein; 11g carbohydrate; 4g dietary fiber, sodium 267 mg

Baked Sole in Creamy Curry Sauce

Prep Time: 5 minutes
Cooking Time: 30 minutes
Serves: 1

Ingredients:
- ✓ 1/2 cup plain yogurt
- ✓ 1/4 cup mayonnaise
- ✓ 1/2 tablespoon lemon juice
- ✓ 1/2 teaspoon curry powder
- ✓ 1-pound sole fillets

Steps:
1) To make the sauce, mix everything except the sole fillets.
2) Spray an 8" x 8" baking dish with non-tick cooking spray. Spread the fillets

with some sauce, rolling them up and down to thoroughly coat them. Place in the baking dish.

3) Spoon the rest of the sauce over and around the fish. Bake at 350 degrees F. for 30 minutes.

Nutritional Breakdown: 296 calories; 19g fat;30g protein; 2g carbohydrate; 0g dietary fiber, sodium 466 mg

Tilapia in Brown Butter

Prep Time: 5 minutes
Cooking Time: 20 minutes
Serves: 1

Ingredients:

- ✓ 1/4 stick butter
- ✓ 1/2-pound tilapia fillets
- ✓ juice and zest of 1 lemon
- ✓ fresh thyme to taste (optional)
- ✓ salt and pepper to taste
- ✓ paprika to taste

Steps:
1) Pre-heat oven to 450 degrees F. Put butter in a 9" x 13" baking dish and place

in the hot oven until the butter is melted and browned.

2) Reduce heat to 400 degrees. Place the fish in the hot butter and bake for 15 minutes.
3) Turn the fillets and baste with the pan juices.
4) Sprinkle the fillet with lemon juice, lemon zest, thyme, salt, pepper and paprika.
5) Bake for 5 more minutes.

Nutritional Breakdown: 393 calories; 25g fat;41g protein; 1g carbohydrate; 0g dietary fiber, sodium 199 mg

Pan Barbecued Sea Bass

Prep Time: 2 minutes
Cooking Time: 10 minutes
Serves: 1

Ingredients:

- ✓ 1/2-pound sea bass fillet
- ✓ 1 tablespoon classic barbeque rub
- ✓ 2 slices bacon
- ✓ 1 tablespoon lemon juice

Steps:

1) Sprinkle both sides of the fillet with the b-b-q rub.
2) Spray a large skillet with non-stick cooking spray and place over a low heat.
3) Using scissors to cut small portions of bacon directly into the skillet.
4) After 2 minutes, add the fish fillets.
5) After 4 minutes, flip the fish over, stirring the bacon. Cook for a further 4 minutes.
6) Take the fillet off the heat and put on a serving plate. Top with the browned bacon. Pour on the lemon juice.

Nutritional Breakdown: 202 calories; 7g fat;31g protein; 2g carbohydrate; 0g dietary fiber, sodium 226 mg

Note: Steaming is the gentlest way to cook vegetables without losing nutrients, a vital consideration on a keto diet. Check out the best price on steamers here: **http://amzn.to/1VadF5k**

Orange Tequila Steak

Prep Time: 5 minutes (plus overnight refrigeration)
Cooking Time: 12 minutes
Serves: 1

Ingredients:

- ✓ 1/2-pound beef steak
- ✓ 2 cloves garlic
- ✓ 1/4 cup lemon juice
- ✓ 1/4 cup lime juice
- ✓ 1 shot tequila
- ✓ 1 teaspoon chili powder
- ✓ 1/2 tablespoon Splenda
- ✓ 1 teaspoon dried oregano
- ✓ 1 1/2 tablespoons olive oil
- ✓ 1/4 teaspoon orange extract

Steps:
1) Mix all the ingredients except the steak in a re-sealable bag and mix together. Add the steak and turn the bag to fully cover it. Place in the refrigerator to marinade overnight.
2) Pour the marinade out into a bowl.
3) Grill the steak for 12 minutes (6 mins per side) on medium heat.
4) Baste at least 2 times during cooking.

Nutritional Breakdown: 560 calories; 46g fat;26g protein; 6g carbohydrate; 1g dietary fiber, sodium 576 mg

Smoky Marinated Steak

Prep Time: 5 minutes (plus overnight refrigeration)
Cooking Time: 12 minutes
Serves: 1

Ingredients:

- ✓ 1/2-pound T-bone steak
- ✓ 1/2 tablespoon liquid smoke flavoring
- ✓ 1 teaspoon salt
- ✓ 1 clove garlic, crushed
- ✓ 1 dash pepper
- ✓ 1 teaspoon olive oil
- ✓ 1/8 teaspoon onion powder
- ✓ 1/4 cup water

Steps:
1) Mix all the ingredients except the steak in a re-sealable bag and mix together. Add the steak and turn the bag to fully cover it. Place in the refrigerator to marinade overnight.
2) Pour the marinade out in a bowl. Broil the steak for six minutes on each side.

Baste half way through, using the reserved marinade.
3) Top with sautéed mushrooms.

Nutritional Breakdown: 276 calories; 20g fat;23g protein; 1g carbohydrate; 0g dietary fiber, sodium 398 mg

Bacon Chili Burgers

Prep Time: 5 minutes (plus overnight refrigeration)
Cooking Time: 12 minutes
Serves: 1

Ingredients:
- ✓ 1-thick slice bacon
- ✓ 1/2 teaspoon extra virgin oil
- ✓ 1/2 pound ground chuck steak
- ✓ 1/4 small onion, chopped
- ✓ 1/2 teaspoon chili garlic paste
- ✓ lettuce leaves

Steps:
1) Place the ground chuck, onion and chili garlic paste in a mixing bowl.
2) Crumble the bacon into the bowl. Mix together with your hands.
3) Form the mixture into a burger.

4) Cook the burgers for six minutes on an electric table-top grill.
5) Sere with lettuce leaves as burger buns.

Nutritional Breakdown: 485 calories; 38g fat;31g protein; 2g carbohydrate; 0g dietary fiber, sodium 268 mg

Hamburger Curry

Prep Time: 5 minutes (plus overnight refrigeration)
Cooking Time: 41 minutes
Serves: 1

Ingredients:

- ✓ 1/2-pound ground beef
- ✓ 1/4 cup chopped onion
- ✓ 1/2 teaspoon curry powder
- ✓ 1 clove garlic
- ✓ 4 ounces tomato sauce
- ✓ 1/4 cup water
- ✓ 1 teaspoon lemon juice
- ✓ 1/4 head cauliflower

Steps:
1) Brown the ground beef in a skillet with medium heat.

2) Pour off the fat and add in the onions, curry, garlic, tomato sauce and water. Cover, turn down the heat and allow to simmer for 30 minutes. Then add the lemon juice and let it simmer for 5 more minutes.
3) Place the cauliflower in a food processor and shred thoroughly. Place in a microwavable casserole dish and microwave for 6 minutes on high with a tablespoon of water.
4) Serve the curry over the cauli-rice.

Nutritional Breakdown: 578 calories; 46g fat;30g protein; 12g carbohydrate; 3g dietary fiber, sodium 288 mg

Note: A Zester will allow you to quickly add the zest of fruits like lemons, limes and oranges to your recipes. Check out the best deal on zesters here: **http://amzn.to/1R9HpIJ**

Cranberry Meatballs

Prep Time: 5 minutes (plus overnight refrigeration)
Cooking Time: 35 minutes
Serves: 1

Ingredients:

- ✓ 1-pound ground beef
- ✓ 1 egg
- ✓ 1/2 teaspoon salt
- ✓ 1/4 teaspoon pepper
- ✓ 1/2 teaspoon dry mustard
- ✓ 4 ounces tomato sauce
- ✓ 1/2 cup cranberries
- ✓ 1 tablespoon Splenda
- ✓ 1/2 tablespoon lime juice
- ✓ 1/4 cup water

Steps:

1) Combine the ground beef, egg, minced onion, salt, pepper and mustard in a large bowl. Mix together by hand. Form into meatballs about 11/2 inches in diameter.
2) Pulse all the other ingredients in a food processor so that the cranberries are finely chopped.
3) Brown the meatballs in a skillet over a medium heat. Pour off the fat and add the sauce. Reduce the heat and simmer for 30 minutes.

Nutritional Breakdown: 577 calories; 47g fat;31g protein; 8g carbohydrate; 2g dietary fiber, sodium 431 mg

Thai Beef Lettuce Wraps

Prep Time: 5 minutes (plus overnight refrigeration)
Cooking Time: 15 minutes
Serves: 1

Ingredients:

- ✓ 1/2-pound ground round
- ✓ 1/2 teaspoon red pepper flakes
- ✓ 1/4 cup chopped onions
- ✓ 1 clove garlic
- ✓ 1 medium yellow pepper, diced
- ✓ 1/8 cup lemon juice
- ✓ 1 teaspoon chopped fresh mint
- ✓ 1 teaspoon beef bouillon granules
- ✓ 1/2 head cauliflower, shredded
- ✓ 1 tablespoon fish sauce
- ✓ 1 tablespoon soy sauce
- ✓ 1/4 cup chopped peanuts
- ✓ 1/4 cucumber diced small
- ✓ 4 lettuce leaves

Steps:

1) Brown and crumble the ground round and pepper flakes in a large skillet under a medium heat. Spoon off the fat after browning.

2) Add the onion, garlic, pepper, lemon juice, mint and beef bouillon granules. Mix thoroughly. Simmer on low for 6 minutes.
3) Shred the cauliflower in a food processor. Place in a microwavable casserole dish and microwave for 6 minutes on high with a tablespoon of water.
4) Drain the cauli-rice then add in the beef mixture, followed by the fish and soy sauce. Stir to mix together.
5) Serve on lettuce leaves and sprinkle with peanuts and cucumber.

Nutritional Breakdown: 413 calories; 29g fat;28g protein; 12g carbohydrate; 3g dietary fiber, sodium 421 mg

Chile Con Carne

Prep Time: 5 minutes (plus overnight refrigeration)
Cooking Time: 35 minutes
Serves: 1

Ingredients:

- ✓ 1/2-pound lean ground beef
- ✓ 1/2 14.5 ounce can stewed tomatoes

- ✓ 1/2 15 oz. can black soy bean
- ✓ 1/2 medium yellow onion, diced
- ✓ 1 tablespoon chili powder
- ✓ 1/2 teaspoon salt
- ✓ 1/4 teaspoon cumin
- ✓ 1/4 teaspoon red pepper
- ✓ 1 bay leaf
- ✓ 1 whole clove garlic
- ✓ Toppings:
- ✓ Diced Onion
- ✓ Sour Cream
- ✓ Shredded cheddar cheese

Steps:

1) Brown the ground beef in a saucepan on a medium heat. Drain off excess fat.
2) Add the remaining ingredients. Cover and simmer on a low heat for one hour. Check after 30 minutes and add water if needed.
3) Remove bay leaf. Serve warm with diced onion, sour cream, and shredded cheddar cheese as toppings.

Nutritional Breakdown: 457 calories; 30g fat;31g protein; 19g carbohydrate; 10g dietary fiber, sodium 466 mg

Marinated Pot Roast

Prep Time: 5 minutes (plus overnight refrigeration)
Cooking Time: 75 minutes
Serves: 1

Ingredients:

- ✓ 1 small turnip
- ✓ 1 stalk celery
- ✓ 1/4 small onion
- ✓ 1/2 cup carrot/zucchini/cauliflower/pepper (depends on personal taste), cut into bite size pieces
- ✓ 1/2 pound London broil
- ✓ 1/2 cup Italian dressing

Steps:

1) Chop up the celery, turnip and onion into small pieces.
2) Place all the vegetables and meat into an oven bag. Mix up with the Italian dressing. Place in refrigerator to marinate overnight.
3) Bake at 350 degrees F. for 75 minutes.

Nutritional Breakdown: 668 calories; 55g fat;29g protein; 14g carbohydrate; 3g dietary fiber, sodium 483 mg

Ginger Sesame Pork

Prep Time: 35 minutes
Cooking Time: 5 minutes
Serves: 1

Ingredients:
- ✓ 3 ounces boneless pork loin
- ✓ 1/4 tablespoon grated ginger
- ✓ 1/2 teaspoons soy sauce
- ✓ 1/8 teaspoon Splenda
- ✓ 1/2 teaspoons toasted sesame oil
- ✓ 1/2 scallions, sliced, including the crisp part of the green
- ✓ 1/2 tablespoon dry sherry
- ✓ 1/2 clove garlic, crushed
- ✓ 1/2 tablespoon peanut oil

Steps:
1) Slice the boneless pork as thinly as you can.
2) Mix all ingredients, except the pork, in a bowl. Add the pork, stir to coat, and let it marinate for 30 minutes.
3) Heat the oil in a skillet. Add the pork and marinade and stir fry for 4-5 minutes, until the meat is thoroughly cooked.

Nutritional Breakdown: 393 calories; 25g fat;31g protein; 5g carbohydrate; 1g dietary fiber, sodium 395 mg

Island Pork Steaks

Prep Time: 50 minutes
Cooking Time: 20 minutes
Serves: 1

Ingredients:

- ✓ 1/2-pound pork shoulder steaks
- ✓ 1 teaspoon ground allspice
- ✓ 1/4 teaspoon ground nutmeg
- ✓ 1/2 teaspoon dried thyme
- ✓ 1/8 teaspoon cayenne
- ✓ 1 tablespoon olive oil
- ✓ 1/4 cup chopped onion
- ✓ 1/4 cup lime juice
- ✓ 1/4 cup chicken broth
- ✓ 1 teaspoon Splenda
- ✓ 1 clove garlic minced

Steps:
1) Mix together the allspice, nutmeg, thyme and cayenne. Coat both sides of the pork with this mixture. Leave to marinade for 30-45 minutes.

2) Heat the olive oil in a large skillet under a medium heat. Add in the pork steaks. Cook for 6-7 minutes on each side. Remove to a plate.

3) Put the onion in the skillet and sauté under a medium heat. Add the like juice, chicken broth, Splenda and garlic. Turn up the heat, and boil the sauce until it is reduced by a half. Pour over the pork and serve.

Nutritional Breakdown: 503 calories; 40g fat;30g protein; 5g carbohydrate; 1g dietary fiber, sodium 407 mg

Note: A food saver is a vacuum sealing devise that will keep your food fresher for longer. It will allow you to prepare vegetables and meats ahead of time. Check out the best deal on food savers here: **http://amzn.to/1UokjGa**

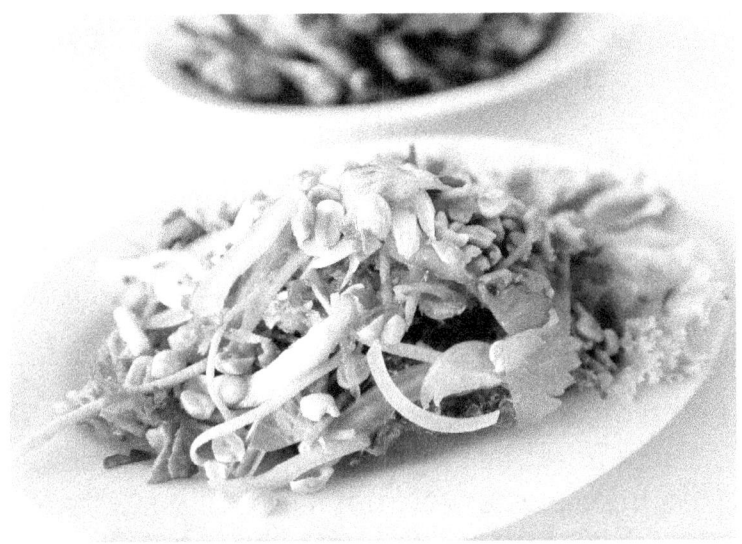

Salads

Asian Chicken Salad

Prep Time: 5 minutes
Cooking Time: 50 minutes (chicken)
Serves: 1

Ingredients:

- ✓ 1 c. carrots, shredded
- ✓ 1/2 c. cabbage, shredded
- ✓ 1/2 c. kale, chopped
- ✓ 1/2 tablespoon black sesame seeds
- ✓ 1/4 jalapeno pepper; ribbed, seeded and finely diced

✓ 2 oz. boneless skinless chicken breast, cooked and shredded
✓ juiceless of half a lime
✓ 1/8 c. soy sauce

Steps:
1) In a bowl, combine carrots, cabbage, kale, sesame seeds, jalapeno and chicken.
2) In another bowl, whisk together lime juice, soy sauce, hot sauce and stevia.
3) Toss the dressing with the salad and serve.

Nutritional Breakdown: 103 calories; 2g fat;4g protein; 19g carbohydrate; 11g dietary fiber, sodium 488 mg

Chef's Salad

Prep Time: 5 minutes
Cooking Time: 0 minutes
Serves: 1

Ingredients:

✓ 1 cup romaine lettuce, torn into bite size pieces
✓ 1 oz. prewashed spinach, trimmed

- ✓ 2 ounces turkey breast or chicken breast, cut into strips
- ✓ 1 ounce baked ham, cut into strips
- ✓ 1 oz. Swiss cheese, cut into strips
- ✓ 1 hard boiled egg, peeled and quartered
- ✓ favorite salad dressing

Steps:

1) Combine the lettuce, spinach, turkey, ham, cheese and eggs in a large salad bowl. Add just enough dressing to bind the ingredients together. Lightly blend.

Nutritional Breakdown: 293 calories; 16g fat;32g protein; 3g carbohydrate; 2.1g dietary fiber, sodium 407 mg

Cob Chicken Salad

Prep Time: 30 minutes
Cooking Time: 0 minutes
Serves: 1

Ingredients:

- ✓ 1/8 cup extra virgin olive oil
- ✓ 1/8 balsamic vinegar
- ✓ 1/2 teaspoon
- ✓ 1/4 teaspoon coarse salt

- ✓ 1/4 teaspoon freshly ground pepper
- ✓ 2 cups romaine lettuce, torn into bite size pieces
- ✓ 1 cooked chicken breast halves, thinly sliced
- ✓ 2 sliced crispy bacon, crumbled
- ✓ 1 hard boiled egg quartered
- ✓ 2 ounces preferred cheese, crumbled
- ✓ 1/4 avocado, peeled and diced (optional)

Steps:

1) Prepare the balsamic vinaigrette by combining the olive oil, vinegar, mustard, salt and pepper in a jar. Shake until well blended. Refrigerate until needed.
2) To prepare the cobb salad, place the lettuce, chicken, bacon, eggs, cheese an optional avocado in a large salad bowl and lightly toss.
3) Add enough balsamic vinaigrette to make the lettuce leaves glisten. Toss the salad again.

Nutritional Breakdown: 777 calories; 60g fat;48g protein; 10g carbohydrate; 4g dietary fiber, sodium 531 mg

Note: A mandolin is a useful tool for slicing, ribboning and julienning your vegetables quickly and easily. Find the best mandolin deal here: <u>http://amzn.to/1Tozewt</u>

Fresh Flounder Salad

Prep Time: 20 minutes
Cooking Time: 8 minutes
Serves: 1

Ingredients:

- ✓ 1 1/4 teaspoon extra virgin olive oil
- ✓ 1/4-pound flounder
- ✓ 1/4 cup finely sliced celery
- ✓ 1 green onion, thinly sliced
- ✓ 1 tablespoon chopped fresh dill
- ✓ 1/8 cup mayonnaise
- ✓ 1/4 teaspoon coarse salt
- ✓ 1/4 teaspoon freshly ground pepper
- ✓ 1 cup red leaf lettuce
- ✓ 1 sprigs of fresh dill, for garnish (optional)

Steps:
1) Heat a large non-stick skillet over medium heat for 2 minutes. Add the olive oil and swirl the pan to coat the bottom evenly.

2) Add the flounder and sauté for 3 minutes on each side.
3) Transfer the flounder to a large bowl and allow it to cool for 10 minutes.
4) Break up the flounder and add the celery, green, onions and dill. Add just enough mayonnaise to bind the ingredients together. Season with salt and pepper and lightly blend.
5) Serve by making a bed with lettuce and mound the flounder salad in the center. Garnish with a sprig of dill.

Nutritional Breakdown: 350 calories; 27g fat;22g protein; 3g carbohydrate; 2g dietary fiber, sodium 503 mg

Italian Beef Salad

Prep Time: 5 minutes (plus overnight refrigeration)
Cooking Time: 45 minutes
Serves: 1

Ingredients:

- ✓ 1/2 tablespoon garlic red wine vinegar
- ✓ 1/2 teaspoon Dijon mustard
- ✓ 1/4 teaspoon dried basil
- ✓ 1/4 oregano leaves

- ✓ 1/4 coarse salt
- ✓ 1/4 freshly ground pepper
- ✓ 1/4 cup extra virgin olive oil
- ✓ 2 ounces beef (your preferred kind)
- ✓ 2 cups romaine lettuce, torn into large bite size pieces
- ✓ 1/4-pound provolone cheese, cubed
- ✓ 1/8 cup thinly sliced red onion

Steps:

1) To make the Italian Vinaigrette, combine the vinegar, mustard, basil, oregano, salt and pepper in a bowl and blend well. Whisk in the olive oil until well mixed.
2) Put the beef in a re-sealable plastic bag and add ¼ cup of the vinaigrette. Turn to coat all over. Seal the bag and refrigerate overnight.
3) Refrigerate the remainder of the vinaigrette until needed.
4) Pre-heat the oven to 400 degrees F. Remove the beef from the marinade and place it in a shallow pan. Bake for 40-45 minutes. Allow the beef to come to room temperature before cutting it into thin slices.
5) To serve, combine the lettuce, beef, cheese and onion in a large bowl and lightly toss. Add the remaining vinaigrette and toss well.

Nutritional Breakdown: 490 calories; 42g fat;25g protein; 4g carbohydrate; 2g dietary fiber, sodium 442 mg

Savory Spinach Salad with Steak and Blue Cheese

Prep Time: 5 minutes
Cooking Time: 8 minutes
Serves: 1

Ingredients:

- ✓ 1 cup pre washed spinach
- ✓ 1/2 pound southwestern rubbed flank steak
- ✓ 1 ounce of your favorite cheese, crumbled
- ✓ 1/4 red pepper cut up
- ✓ 1/2 green onion, finely sliced
- ✓ 1 tablespoon Balsamic Vinaigrette

Steps:
1) Combine the spinach, flank steak, cheese, red pepper and green onions in a large bowl. Add just enough balsamic vinaigrette to make the spinach leaves glisten. Toss well.

Nutritional Breakdown: 407 calories; 22g fat;44g protein; 7g carbohydrate; 3g dietary fiber, sodium 789 mg

Mixed Baby Greens with Blue Cheese and Walnuts

Prep Time: 5 minutes
Cooking Time: 0 minutes
Serves: 1

Ingredients:
- ✓ 1 tablespoon white wine vinegar
- ✓ 1/2 tablespoon Dijon mustard
- ✓ 1/2 tablespoon fresh lemon juice
- ✓ 1/4 teaspoon coarse salt
- ✓ 1/8 teaspoon freshly ground pepper
- ✓ 1/4 cup canola oil
- ✓ 2 cups mixed baby greens
- ✓ 1/4 small red onion, thinly sliced
- ✓ 1/4 cup crumbled cheese
- ✓ 1/4 cup chopped walnuts

Steps:
1) To make the white wine vinaigrette, whisk the vinegar, mustard, lemon juice, salt, and pepper in a bowl and mix well. Gradually whisk in the canola oil until everything is thoroughly blended.

2) To serve, combine the mixed baby greens, red onion, cheese and. walnuts in a salad bowl. Add enough white wine vinaigrette to make the lettuce leaves glisten and gently toss.

Nutritional Breakdown: 251 calories; 23g fat;7g protein; 5g carbohydrate; 2g dietary fiber, sodium 470 mg

Romaine Salad with Romano Cheese

Prep Time: 5 minutes
Cooking Time: 0 minutes
Serves: 1

Ingredients:

- ✓ 1 tablespoon fresh lemon juice
- ✓ 1 egg
- ✓ 1/4 teaspoon coarse salt
- ✓ 1/4 teaspoon dried oregano leaves
- ✓ 1/8 teaspoon dried mint leaves
- ✓ 1/4 cup extra virgin olive oil
- ✓ 2 cups romaine lettuce, torn into generous bite size pieces
- ✓ 1/2 cup freshly grated Romano cheese

Steps:

1) For the Caesar dressing, combine the lemon juice, egg, salt, pepper, oregano, turmeric and mint in a food processor. Pour in the olive oil and blend thoroughly. Refrigerate overnight.
2) To serve, place the lettuce and cheese in a salad bowl and toss vigorously. Coat the lettuce leaves with the Caesar dressing

Nutritional Breakdown: 333 calories; 33g fat;7g protein; 4g carbohydrate; 2g dietary fiber, sodium 406 mg

Note: With a Vegetable Spiralizer you'll be able to make low-carb vegetable spaghetti adding texture and substance to your keto meals. Find the best Spiralizer deal here: http://amzn.to/1W3osiN

Spinach Salad with Maytag Blue Cheese

Prep Time: 5 minutes
Cooking Time: 0 minutes
Serves: 1

Ingredients:

- ✓ 1 cup pre washed spinach
- ✓ 1/2 cup Boston lettuce, torn into generous bite pieces
- ✓ 1/2 green onion, thinly sliced
- ✓ 1 ounce Maytag blue cheese
- ✓ 1 tablespoon balsamic vinaigrette
- ✓ 1/4 red pepper, thinly sliced

Steps:

1) Combine the spinach, lettuce, green onions, and cheese in a large bowl. Add enough Balsamic Vinaigrette to make the leaves glisten.
2) To serve, arrange the salad on a plate and distribute the red pepper strips over it.

Nutritional Breakdown: 242 calories; 23g fat;5g protein; 5g carbohydrate; 2g dietary fiber, sodium 422 mg

Cauliflower Salad

Prep Time: 5 minutes
Cooking Time: 3-4 minutes
Serves: 1

Ingredients:

- ✓ 1 head cauliflower

- ✓ 1 egg, hard boiled and chopped
- ✓ 1/2 celery stalk, finely sliced
- ✓ 1/4 red onion, finely chopped
- ✓ 1/4 c. dill pickles finely chopped
- ✓ 1/2 c. plain Greek yogurt
- ✓ 1 teaspoon dried dill
- ✓ 1 teaspoon garlic powder

Steps:
1) Add about an inch of water to a large, microwave-safe bowl. Add chopped cauliflower to the bowl. Microwave on high for 3-4 minutes.
2) Drain and pat the cauliflower dry and crumble it into a large bowl. Stir in the eggs, celery, onion and pickles.
3) In a separate bowl, whisk together the yogurt, dill, garlic, mustard and pepper. Stir the yogurt mixture into the cauliflower until evenly coated.
4) Serve immediately, or chill in the refrigerator for two hours.

Nutritional Breakdown: 129 calories; 5g fat;12g protein; 5g carbohydrate; 1g dietary fiber, sodium 458 mg

Shrimp and Avocado Salad

Prep Time: 5 minutes (plus 2 hours refrigeration)
Cooking Time: 0 minutes
Serves: 1

Ingredients:

- ✓ 1 tablespoon fresh lime juice
- ✓ 1/2 tablespoon extra virgin olive oil
- ✓ 1/4 c. cilantro, chopped
- ✓ 1/8 teaspoon salt
- ✓ 1/8 teaspoon pepper
- ✓ 1/2 lb. cooked shrimp, peeled and deveined
- ✓ 1/2 avocado, pitted and chopped
- ✓ 1 c. lettuce, chopped

Steps:
1) In a bowl, whisk together lime juice, oil, cilantro, salt and pepper. Toss in the shrimp and refrigerate for 2 hours.
2) Once marinated, toss the shrimp and the remaining dressing with avocado and lettuce. Serve immediately.

Nutritional Breakdown: 330 calories; 20g fat;28g protein; 9g carbohydrate; 3g dietary fiber, sodium 466 mg

Carrot and Edamame Citrus Salad

Prep Time: 7 minutes
Cooking Time: 0 minutes
Serves: 1

Ingredients:

- ✓ 1 carrot peeled and cut into thin matchsticks
- ✓ 1/4 c. frozen shelled edamame, thawed
- ✓ 1/4 c. cilantro, chopped
- ✓ 1/8 c. black sesame seeds
- ✓ 1/8 c. fresh orange juice
- ✓ juice of 1/2 lime
- ✓ 1/2 tablespoon of ginger root, minced
- ✓ 1 teaspoon agave syrup

Steps:
1) In a large bowl, combine carrots, edamame, cilantro and sesame seeds.
2) In a separate bowl, whisk together orange juice, lime juice, ginger, agave, sesame oil, salt and pepper. Steam in grape-seed oil, whisking until well combined.
3) Toss the salad with dressing and slice with the tossed avocado and serve.

Nutritional Breakdown: 503 calories; 40g fat;30g protein; 5g carbohydrate; 1g dietary fiber, sodium 407 mg

Eggplant Salsa Stacks

Prep Time: 30 minutes
Cooking Time: 8 minutes
Serves: 1

Ingredients:

- ✓ 1/2 lb. eggplant
- ✓ 1/2 teaspoon salt
- ✓ 1 egg
- ✓ 1 1/2 oz. parmesan cheese, finely grated
- ✓ 1/4 almond meal
- ✓ 1 clove garlic, minced
- ✓ 1/2 tablespoon vegetable oil
- ✓ 1/4 cup salsa

Steps:
1) Slice the eggplant lengthwise and sprinkle with salt. Let sit for 20 minutes then pat dry.
2) Whisk egg in a bowl.
3) In a separate bowl, combine the cheese, almond meal and garlic.
4) Heat the oil in a skillet. Dip each eggplant slice in egg and then cheese mixture, then place them in the skillet. Cook for 4 minutes each side.

5) Top the cooked eggplant with salsa, then another slice of eggplant. Serve.

Nutritional Breakdown: 337 calories; 23g fat;20g protein; 17g carbohydrate; 11g dietary fiber, sodium 417 mg

<u>Veggie Egg Salad</u>

Prep Time: 5 minutes
Cooking Time: 12 minutes
Serves: 1

Ingredients:

- ✓ 1/8 cup plain Greek yogurt
- ✓ 1/2 teaspoon Dijon mustard
- ✓ 1/8 teaspoon pepper
- ✓ 1/8 teaspoon salt
- ✓ 2 hard boiled eggs
- ✓ 1/8 cup carrot, finely chopped
- ✓ 1/8 cup cucumber, finely chopped
- ✓ 1/8 cup green onions, finely chopped

Steps:
1) In a bowl, combine yogurt, mustard, pepper and salt.
2) Cut each egg in half and remove the yolks. Discard half the yolks

3) Chop the remaining yolks and whites
and stir into the yogurt mixture.
4) Stir in vegetables and serve.

*Nutritional Breakdown: 135 calories; 40g
fat;7g protein; 11g carbohydrate; 7g dietary
fiber, sodium 431 mg*

Creamy Lemon-Lime Smoothie

Prep Time: 30 seconds
Serves: 1

Ingredients:

- ✓ ½ teaspoon fresh lemon juice
- ✓ ½ teaspoon fresh lime juice
- ✓ ½ cup yogurt
- ✓ 1 tablespoon honey
- ✓ several leaves mint

Steps:
1) Blend the juices with the honey and yogurt.
2) Serve with fresh mint leaves

Nutritional Breakdown: 115 calories; 65g fat;20g protein;7g carbohydrate; 3g dietary fiber, sodium 121 mg

Note: High power blenders will, not only allow you to whip up the smoothies in this section; you'll also be able to puree sauces with ease. Check out the best price on quality blenders here: **http://amzn.to/1TkLo7r**

Cranberry Cocoa Smoothie

Prep Time: 45 seconds
Serves: 1
Ingredients:

- ✓ 1 oz. fresh cranberries
- ✓ 100 ml. cocoa milk
- ✓ ¼ teaspoon cinnamon

Steps:
1) Blend the cranberries and filter the mixture using a strainer.
2) Add the cocoa milk and cinnamon.
3) Bend for a further 15 seconds.

Nutritional Breakdown: 80 calories; 13g fat;27g protein;8.9g carbohydrate; 3.4g dietary fiber, sodium 135 mg

Wildberry Smoothie

Prep Time: 50 seconds
Serves: 1

Ingredients:

- ✓ 3oz. fresh or frozen wildberries

- ✓ 2 oz. low fat milk
- ✓ 2 tablespoons mint syrup
- ✓ leaves of mint for garnish

Steps:
1) Put the fruits in the blender together with the leaves of fresh mint and grind well.
2) Add the milk and blend for 30 seconds.

Nutritional Breakdown: 112 calories; 23g fat;17g protein;4.9g carbohydrate; 1.4g dietary fiber, sodium 125 mg

Green Machine Smoothie

Prep Time: 10 minutes
Serves: 1

Ingredients:

- ✓ 1.5 oz. boiled spinach
- ✓ 1.5 oz. boiled broccoli
- ✓ 1.5 oz. boiled asparagus
- ✓ 1.5 oz. boiled courgettes

Steps:
1) Boil the vegetables.
2) Blend the vegetables, adding water to achieve the desired thickness.

Nutritional Breakdown: 140 calories; 8g fat;37g protein;4.5g carbohydrate; 2.4g dietary fiber, sodium 188 mg

Grapefruit Smoothie

Prep Time: 30 seconds
Serves: 1

Ingredients:

- ✓ 1.75 oz. pink grapefruit juice
- ✓ 1.75 oz. yellow grapefruit juice
- ✓ 1.75 oz. orange juice
- ✓ crushed ice - optional

Steps:
1) Mixed the freshly squeezed juices
2) Cover with crushed ice and serve

Nutritional Breakdown: 44 calories; 0.2g fat;0.9g protein;10g carbohydrate; 5.8g dietary fiber, sodium 175 mg

Raspberry Smoothie

Prep Time: 50 seconds
Serves: 1

Ingredients:

- ✓ 1.5 oz. raspberries
- ✓ 4 oz. vanilla milk
- ✓ 1/3 oz. chocolate chips
- ✓ 1 tablespoon protein powder

Steps:
1) Blend the raspberries.
2) Add the milk and protein powder until smooth.
3) Top the chocolate chips when you serve.

Nutritional Breakdown: 312 calories; 58g fat;28g protein;10g carbohydrate; 5.2g dietary fiber, sodium 255 mg

<u>Milk Chocolate Smoothie</u>

Prep Time: 30 seconds
Serves: 1

Ingredients:

- ✓ 4 oz. yogurt
- ✓ 1.5 oz. milk chocolate
- ✓ ½ banana
- ✓ 1 tablespoon coca flavor
- ✓ 0.75 oz. water

Steps:
1) Puree the banana and melted milk chocolate.
2) Add the yogurt and coca flavor and blend for a further 15 seconds.
3) Dilute with water if needed.

Nutritional Breakdown: 510 calories; 78g fat;23g protein;9.8g carbohydrate; 3.4g dietary fiber, sodium 288 mg

Mocha Surprise Smoothie

Prep Time: 5 minutes
Serves: 1

Ingredients:

- ✓ 6 oz. Mocha coffee
- ✓ 2 tablespoon dry cream
- ✓ 3 oz. milk
- ✓ 2 tablespoon cocoa protein
- ✓ crushed ice - optional

Steps:
1) Prepare a strong mocha coffee and blend it with the milk and dry cream for 7-8 minutes.

2) Add the protein powder. Blend for a further 15 seconds.
3) Add ice if desired.

Nutritional Breakdown: 140 calories; 35g fat;19g protein;9g carbohydrate; 1.5g dietary fiber, sodium 312 mg

Dark Chocolate Coconut Smoothie

Prep Time: 60 seconds
Serves: 1

Ingredients:

- ✓ 1.5 oz. dark chocolate 99% cocoa
- ✓ 4 oz. milk
- ✓ 1 tablespoon coconut flakes
- ✓ 1 tablespoon almond flakes

Steps:
1) Melt the chocolate
2) Blend the chocolate and milk for 30 seconds.
3) Top with flakes of coconut and almonds.

Nutritional Breakdown: 340 calories; 49g fat;16.5g protein;9.5g carbohydrate; 2.2g dietary fiber, sodium 251 mg

Busy Bee Banana Smoothie

Prep Time: 30 seconds (plus overnight refrigeration)
Serves: 1

Ingredients:

- ✓ 1 banana
- ✓ 1 cup soy milk
- ✓ ¼ cup rolled oats
- ✓ 1 teaspoon honey
- ✓ pinch of cinnamon

Steps:
1) Place all of the ingredients in the bender bowl and refrigerate overnight.
2) In the morning, blend for 30 seconds.

Nutritional Breakdown: 291 calories; 5.9g fat;15g protein;8.9g carbohydrate; 3.4g dietary fiber, sodium 505 mg

Avocado-Coconut Smoothie

Prep Time: 50 seconds
Serves: 1

Ingredients:

- ✓ 2 slices avocado
- ✓ 2 oz. nonfat cottage cheese
- ✓ 1 tablespoon coconut oil
- ✓ 2.75 oz. water
- ✓ colored coconut flakes

Steps:
1) Peel the avocado carefully, remove the pit and out the flesh in the blender.
2) Add the non-fat cottage cheese, coconut oil and the water.
3) Stir the ingredients in the blender.
4) Top with some colored coconut flakes.

Nutritional Breakdown: 193 calories; 14.7g fat;11.9g protein;3.1g carbohydrate; 1.8g dietary fiber, sodium 251 mg

Veggie Bouquet Smoothie

Prep Time: 50 seconds
Serves: 1

Ingredients:

- ✓ 3 oz. cucumbers
- ✓ 1.5 oz. tomatoes
- ✓ 1 oz. green onion

- ✓ 1 oz. lettuce
- ✓ fresh leaves of parsley

Steps:

1) Wash the vegetables and leave them on a paper towel to dry out.
2) Place all vegetables in a blender and mix for 5-6 minutes.
3) Serve with fresh leaves of parsley

Nutritional Breakdown:63 calories; 2g fat;17g protein;9.8g carbohydrate; 6.9g dietary fiber, sodium 344 mg

<u>Sunshine Smoothie</u>

Prep Time: 30 seconds (plus overnight refrigeration)
Serves: 1

Ingredients:

- ✓ 1/2 cup of chopped pineapple (fresh is best, but tinned will work in a pinch)
- ✓ 1/2 ripe banana
- ✓ 1 kiwi (peeled)
- ✓ 1 cup of baby spinach
- ✓ A small handful of fresh mint
- ✓ 1 cup of coconut milk

Steps:

1) Place all of the ingredients in the bender bowl and refrigerate overnight.
2) In the morning, blend for 30 seconds.

Nutritional Breakdown: 311 calories; 4.1g fat;21g protein;12.3g carbohydrate; 4.1g dietary fiber, sodium 411 mg

Note: A juicer is a handy appliance when you're in a hurry. It will allow you to get your meals in liquid form when you're on the run. Check out the best price on quality juicers here: **http://amzn.to/23XMVoX**

Toxin Terminator Smoothie

Prep Time: 30 seconds (plus overnight refrigeration)
Serves: 1

Ingredients:

- ✓ 1 apple
- ✓ 1 celery stick
- ✓ ½ cucumber
- ✓ handful of spinach
- ✓ handful of kale
- ✓ 1 cup of ice

Steps:
1) Chop the apple, cucumber and celery stick into slices.
2) Place all ingredients in a blender and process for 5-6 minutes.

Nutritional Breakdown: 301 calories; 5g fat;19g protein;9.9g carbohydrate; 5.1g dietary fiber, sodium 422 mg

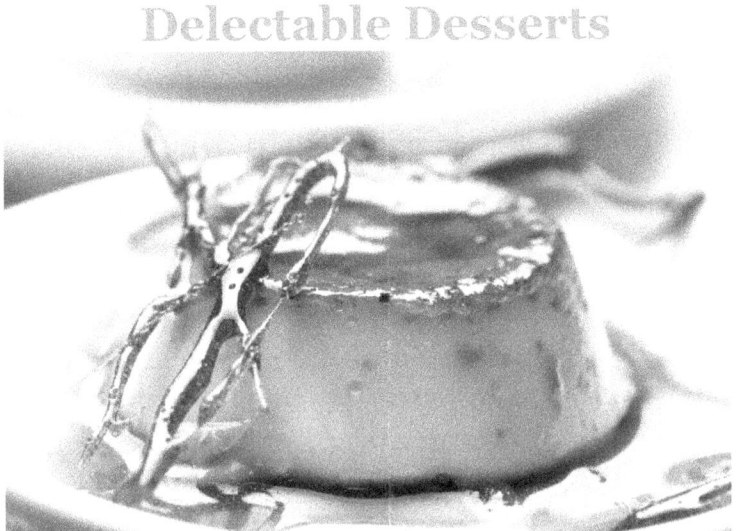

Delectable Desserts

Crème Brulee

Prep Time: 50 minutes
Cooking Time: 20 minutes
Serves: 1

Ingredients:

- ✓ 1/4 cups whipping cream
- ✓ 1/8 teaspoon vanilla
- ✓ 1 large egg yolks
- ✓ 1/8 cup Splenda
- ✓ 1/4 tablespoon dark brown sugar (optional)

Steps:

1) Combine the whipping cream and vanilla in a saucepan. Heat until hot (not boiling). Remove from heat and put on a rack to cool. Then cover and refrigerate for 30 minutes.
2) Pre-heat the oven to 325 degrees F.
3) Place the egg yolk and Splenda in a bowl and mix vigorously. Add the whipping cream mixture and blend well.
4) Place a small strainer over a 4-ounce ramekin. Pour whipping cream mixture almost to the top of the dish.
5) Place the ramekin in a bigger pan and place in the oven. Pour enough water in the pan to come up the sides of the dishes.
6) Cover each crème brulee with plastic wrap and place in the fridge until you are ready to serve them.

Nutritional Breakdown: 332 calories; 34g fat;4g protein; 5g carbohydrate; 0g dietary fiber, sodium 286 mg

Banana, Chocolate Chip and Walnut Muffins

Prep Time: 6 minutes
Cooking Time: 15 minutes
Serves: 1 - (4 muffins)

Ingredients:

- ✓ 3/4 cup vanilla whey protein powder
- ✓ 1/4 cup high-gluten flour
- ✓ 1 1/2 teaspoon baking soda
- ✓ 1/2 teaspoon ground cinnamon
- ✓ 1/2 teaspoon coarse salt
- ✓ 1/2 cup (1 stick) butter, melted
- ✓ 1 cup Splenda
- ✓ 1 cup mashed ripe banana
- ✓ 1/3 cup milk
- ✓ 1 large egg
- ✓ 3/4 cup chopped walnuts

Steps:

1) Pre-heat oven to 350 degrees F. Line muffin tin with paper cup holders.
2) Combine the protein powder, gluten flour, baking flour, baking soda, cinnamon and salt in a bowl and mix vigorously with a whisk.
3) Combine the butter and Splenda in another medium bowl and beat with a whisk for 2 minutes. Add the banana, milk and egg and blend well.
4) Add the dry ingredients and mix with a fork until just blended.
5) Fold in the walnuts and chocolate chips.
6) Spoon the batter into the prepared muffin tin, two thirds full.

7) Bake for 12-15 minutes, until firm to the touch.

Nutritional Breakdown: 234 calories; 17g fat;9g protein; 11g carbohydrate; 1g dietary fiber, sodium 241 mg

Chocolate Chip and Almond Streusel Coffee Cake

Prep Time: 5 minutes
Cooking Time: 20 minutes
Serves: 1

Ingredients:

- ✓ Almond Streusel Topping:
    - o 1/4 cup Splenda
    - o 1/4 cup almond flour
    - o 2 tablespoons butter, well chilled and cut into 8 pieces
    - o 6 tablespoons sliced almonds
    - o 1/4 cup zero-carb chocolate chips
- ✓ Coffeecake:
    - o 3/4 cup vanilla whey protein
    - o 1/4 cup almond flour
    - o 3/4 teaspoon baking soda
    - o 1 egg

Steps:

1) Pre-heat oven to 350 degrees F. Lightly coat a 9-inch round cake pan with a no-stick vegetable spray and dust with almond flour.
2) To make the almond streusel, combine 1/8 cup of Splenda and almond flour in a bowl and mix well. Cut in the butter with a pastry blender. Fold in the almonds and 1/8 cup chocolate chips. Set aside.
3) To make the coffee cake, combine the protein powder, almond flour, baking soda, baking powder, and salt in a medium bowl and blend with a wire whisk. Beat the butter in an electric mixer, and then add the egg. Add ¼ cup of Splenda and beat for 3 minutes. Add the milk and almond extract and blend. Add in the dry ingredients, and finally the chocolate chips.
4) Spoon the batter into the prepared pan and sprinkle the Almond Streusel Topping over the top.
5) Bake for 20 minutes.

Nutritional Breakdown: 256 calories; 20g fat10g protein; 5g carbohydrate; 1g dietary fiber, sodium 166 mg

Macadamia Nut Chocolate Squares

Prep Time: 7 minutes
Cooking Time: 5 minutes
Serves: 1

Ingredients:

- ✓ 2 tablespoons cocoa powder
- ✓ 2 tablespoons sweetener
- ✓ 2 oz. cocoa butter
- ✓ ¼ cup heavy cream

Steps:
1) Melt the cocoa butter in the microwave for 30 seconds.
2) Whisk in the cocoa powder and sweetener.
3) Stir in the macadamia nuts and heavy cream. Mix well.
4) Pour the mixture into a chocolate mold.
5) Allow to cool, the place in the refrigerator to harden.

Nutritional Breakdown: 272 calories;28g fat;3g protein; 3g carbohydrate; 2g dietary fiber, sodium 204

Chocolate Chip and Walnut Shortbread

Prep Time: 4 minutes
Cooking Time: 55 minutes
Serves: 1

Ingredients:

- ✓ 1 cup high-gluten flour
- ✓ 3/4 cup vanilla whey protein
- ✓ 1/2 teaspoon baking soda
- ✓ 1 stick plus 2 tablespoons butter, at room temperature
- ✓ 1/2 cup Splenda
- ✓ 1/2 teaspoon powdered white stevia
- ✓ 1 cup finely chopped walnuts
- ✓ 1 cup zero carbs chocolate chips

Steps:

1) Pre-heat oven to 350 degrees F.
2) Combine the gluten flour, protein powder and baking soda in a bowl and blend with a wire whisk.
3) Put the butter, Splenda and Stevia in a blender and process for 3 minutes. Add the walnuts and blend well.
4) Add the dry ingredients, including the chocolate chips, and mix on a medium speed. Mix until the dough begins to stick together.
5) Press the dough into the prepared pan. Bake for 45-50 minutes.

6) Cool for 15 minutes and then cut into bars.

Nutritional Breakdown: 229 calories; 18g fat;7g protein; 7g carbohydrate; 0g dietary fiber, sodium 45 mg

Ultimate Cheesecake

Prep Time: 25 minutes (plus several hours cooling in refrigerator)
Cooking Time: 60 minutes
Serves: 2 - (1/2 of a small cheesecake)

Ingredients:

- ✓ 1/2 cup walnuts
- ✓ 3 package (8 ounces each) cream cheese, at room temperature
- ✓ 3/4 cups Splenda
- ✓ 1 teaspoon powdered white stevia
- ✓ 4 large eggs
- ✓ 1 1/2 teaspoons vanilla extract

Steps:
1) Pre-heat oven to 350 degrees F. Lightly coat a 9-inch spring form pan with a non-stick vegetable spray.
2) To make the walnut crust, crush the walnuts in a food processor, then press

the walnuts on the bottom of the prepared pan. Bake for 5 minutes.

3) Take the pan out of the oven and set aside to cool.

4) To make the filling, put the crème cheese, ¼ cup of Splenda, in a blender and process for 3 minutes.

5) Add the eggs and ½ teaspoon of vanilla and bet well. On medium speed, add the whipping cream and beat for 2 minutes.

6) Pour the batter into the pan. Place the pan into a larger pan and put in the oven. Pour enough hot water into the pan to come halfway up the pan. Bake for 45 minutes.

7) To make the sour cream topping, combine the sour cream, 1/2 tablespoon Splenda, and ¼ teaspoon vanilla in a small bowl and blend well.

8) Take the cheesecake out of the oven, and allow it to cool for 5 minutes. Spread sour cream topping over top of the cheesecake. Bake for 5 minutes.

9) Leave in the oven for an hour and then refrigerate for several hours before serving.

Nutritional Breakdown: 320 calories; 30g fat;8g protein; 5g carbohydrate; 0g dietary fiber, sodium 202 mg

Chocolate Dipped Shortbread

Prep Time: 10 minutes (plus several hours cooling in refrigerator)
Cooking Time: 12 minutes
Serves: 1

Ingredients:
- ✓ 10 to 12 cookies
- ✓ 1/2 cup (or more) finely ground walnuts or pecans
- ✓ 1 1/2 cups high-gluten flour
- ✓ 1/2 cup vanilla whey protein powder
- ✓ 1/2 teaspoon baking soda
- ✓ 1 cup (2 sticks) butter, at room temperature
- ✓ 1/2 cup Splenda
- ✓ 1 teaspoon powdered white stevia
- ✓ 1 teaspoon vanilla extract
- ✓ 5 to 6 ounces Darrell Lea sugar free milk chocolate or favorite sugar free chocolate, coarsely chopped

Steps:
1) Pre-heat oven to 350 degrees F. Line a baking sheet with parchment paper. Line another baking sheet with a piece of waxed paper. Place the walnuts in a small dish. Set aside.

2) Combine the gluten flour, protein powder, and baking soda in a bowl and mix vigorously.

3) Place the butter, Splenda and Stevia in the bowl of an electric mixer and beat on medium-high for 3 minutes. Add the vanilla and blend well.

4) Add the dry ingredients and beat on medium-low until dough sticks together.

5) Roll the dough into 2-inch logs and place them on the parchment lined baking sheet, an inch apart.

6) Bake for 8-10 minutes. Cool completely.

7) For the chocolate topping, melt the chocolate for 30 seconds in the microwave.

8) Dip the end of each cookie in the chocolate, then roll the dipped end in the walnuts.

9) Place the cookies on the waxed paper-lined cookie sheet and refrigerate until the chocolate has set.

Nutritional Breakdown: 42 calories; 3.5g fat; 1g protein; 2g carbohydrate; 0g dietary fiber, sodium 11 mg

Pie Crust

Prep Time: 5 minutes

Cooking Time: 0 minutes
Serves: 1

Ingredients:

- ✓ ½ cup almond meal
- ✓ 1/3 cup rice protein
- ✓ ¼ cup gluten, wheat
- ✓ 1 pinch baking soda
- ✓ ½ teaspoon salt
- ✓ 1/3 cup coconut oil
- ✓ 1 tablespoon butter
- ✓ 3 tablespoons ice water

Steps:

1) Put the almond meal, rice protein, gluten, baking powder, and salt in a food processor. Add the coconut oil and butter and pulse until you get a mealy texture.
2) Add a tablespoon of ice water, then pulse the food briefly. Do this two more times.
3) Place the dough in a 9-inch pie plate and press into place evenly across the bottom and sides.

Nutritional Breakdown: 194 calories; 15g fat;15g protein; 3g carbohydrate; 1g dietary fiber, sodium 214 mg

Strawberry Cheese Pie

Prep Time: 25 minutes (plus several hours cooling in refrigerator)
Cooking Time: 15 minutes
Serves: 1

Ingredients:

- ✓ 8 oz. Neufchatel cheese, softened
- ✓ 2 tablespoons heavy cream
- ✓ 11/2 tablespoon Splenda
- ✓ ½ teaspoon vanilla extract
- ✓ Pie crust, pre-baked (see previous recipe)
- ✓ 1 pound frozen, unsweetened strawberries
- ✓ 1 cup water
- ✓ 2 tablespoons lemon juice
- ✓ 2 teaspoons unflavored gelatin

Steps:
1) Place the Neufchatel cheese, heavy cream, ½ the Splenda and vanilla until it is very smooth and fluffy.
2) Smooth the mixture over your pre-baked pie shell.
3) Put the strawberries, water, the rest of the Splenda, and lemon juice in a

saucepan. Bring to the boil then turn down to low and let it simmer.

4) Mash the strawberries with a whisk. Sprinkle the gelatin over the strawberry mixture. Turn off the heat and let the mixture cool.

5) Spoon the strawberry layer over the cream cheese layer. Place the pie in the refrigerator for several hours before serving.

Nutritional Breakdown: 307 calories; 22g fat;20g protein; 10g carbohydrate; 2g dietary fiber, sodium 519 mg

Strawberry Ice Cream

Prep Time: 25 minutes (plus several hours cooling in refrigerator)
Cooking Time: 15 minutes
Serves: 1

Ingredients:

- ✓ 1 pound frozen, unsweetened strawberries
- ✓ 4 cups heavy cream
- ✓ ½ teaspoon liquid stevia

Steps:

1) Place all the ingredients in your food processor and bend until the berries are completely ground. Serve immediately.

Nutritional Breakdown: 430 calories; 44g fat;3g protein; 8g carbohydrate; 1g dietary fiber, sodium 288 mg

Crème Polynesienne

Prep Time: 25 minutes
Cooking Time: 0 minutes
Serves: 1

Ingredients:

- ✓ ¾ cup unsweetened coconut milk
- ✓ 2 egg yolks
- ✓ 18 drops liquid stevia (vanilla)
- ✓ ½ teaspoon vanilla extract

Steps:
1) Combine all ingredients in a double boiler over hot water and a lo3 heat. Whisk well to thoroughly combine.
2) Continue whisking until the custard thickens. This will take up to 25 minutes.
3) Remove from heat, cool and chill.

Nutritional Breakdown: 249 calories; 25g fat;5g protein; 3g carbohydrate; 0g dietary fiber, sodium 367 mg

Almond Flour Lemon Pound Cake

Prep Time: 20 minutes
Cooking Time: 50 minutes
Serves: 1

Ingredients:

- ✓ 1 cup almond meal
- ✓ ¼ teaspoon Stevia
- ✓ ½ teaspoon baking soda
- ✓ ½ teaspoon salt
- ✓ ½ cup butter
- ✓ ½ cup Splenda
- ✓ 1 tablespoon lemon zest
- ✓ ½ tablespoon lemon juice
- ✓ 3 large eggs
- ✓ ½ teaspoon vanilla extract
- ✓ 1 tablespoon oat flour

Steps:

1) Heat oven to 350 degrees F. Grease a 9" x 5" loaf pan with a tablespoon of butter and dust with a tablespoon of oat flour.

2) Place the almond meal, Stevia, baking powder and salt in a bowl and mix vigorously. Set aside.

3) In a microwave safe bowl, microwave the butter, covered with plastic wrap on high until melted.

4) Process Splenda and zest in a food processor until combined, then add lemon juice, eggs and vanilla. Add the melted butter through the feed tube slowly.

5) Pour mixture to a bowl. Sift the flour mixture over the egg mixture in three steps, whisking gently after each step.

6) Pour the batter into the pan, baking for 15 minutes. Then reduce oven temperature to 325 degrees and continue baking until done (approx. 35 minutes). Cool in the pan for 10 minutes and then place on a wire rack.

Nutritional Breakdown: 292 calories; 27g fat;6g protein; 6g carbohydrate; 2g dietary fiber, sodium 499 mg

Whipped Topping

Prep Time: 3 minutes
Cooking Time: 0 minutes
Serves: 1

Ingredients:

- ✓ 1 cup heavy cream, well chilled
- ✓ 1 tablespoon sugar-free instant pudding powder (vanilla)

Steps:

1) Whip the ingredients together until the cream is stiff.

Nutritional Breakdown: 188 calories; 32g fat;1g protein; 1g carbohydrate; 0g dietary fiber, sodium 194 mg

<u>Strawberry Fluff</u>

Prep Time: 4 minutes
Cooking Time: 0 minutes
Serves: 1

Ingredients:

- ✓ 2 oz. cream cheese, softened
- ✓ ¼ pack sugar-free strawberry gelatin
- ✓ 1 batch whipped topping
- ✓ chopped nuts

Steps:

1) 1.Use a mixer to beat the cheese until creamy.
2) Beat in the gelatin powder.
3) Fold in the whipped topping and the nuts.
4) Serve immediately or chilled, according to your preference.

Nutritional Breakdown: 338 calories; 34g fat;5g protein; 4g carbohydrate; 0g dietary fiber, sodium 344 mg

Peanut Butter Dough Ice Cream

Prep Time: 4 minutes
Cooking Time: 0 minutes
Serves: 1

Ingredients:

- ✓ ½ packet unflavored, unsweetened gelatin
- ✓ ½ cup hot water
- ✓ 1/2 teaspoon peanut butter extract
- ✓ ½ teaspoon vanilla extract
- ✓ ¾ cup heavy cream
- ✓ ¼ cup Splenda
- ✓ ¼ cup liquid sweetener
- ✓ 1/8 cup egg white protein
- ✓ 1/8 cup natural peanut butter

Steps:
1) Sprinkle gelatin over hot water and let it set for a minute. Stir until gelatin is dissolved.
2) In a food processor combine the Splenda, sweetener, egg protein, gelatin water and peanut butter. Mix well.
3) Cool for 30 minutes.
4) Pour into an ice-cream maker, following the manufacturer's instructions.

Nutritional Breakdown: 435 calories; 40g fat;13g protein; 6g carbohydrate; 0g dietary fiber, sodium 294 mg

Conclusion

The Ketogenic Diet overview and recipes presented have provided you with the tools to embark on the most effective weight loss and general health diet that has yet been created. We encourage you to embrace it, to live it and to love it.

Take the recipes that we have laid out and use them to create mouth watering, fulfilling and weight reducing meals for yourself and your family.

Most importantly, stick to the Keto way of eating. You've spent all of your life up until now stumbling in the dark when it comes to nutrition. Now that you've found the light, cherish it, for it will serve you for the rest of your days.

References

1) A high-monounsaturated-fat/low-carbohydrate diet improves peripheral insulin sensitivity in non-insulin-dependent diabetic patients. - 1992
   a. Parillo, M. et al., 1992.
   b. Metabolism, 41(12), pp.1373–1378.
   c. Available at: http://www.ncbi.nlm.nih.gov/pubmed/1461145

2) Therapeutic role of low-carbohydrate ketogenic diet in diabetes. - 2009
   a. Al-Khalifa, A. et al., 2009.
   b. Nutrition (Burbank, Los Angeles County, Calif.), 25(11-12), pp.1177–1185.
   c. Available at: http://www.ncbi.nlm.nih.gov/pubmed/19818281/

3) Meta-analysis of prospective cohort studies evaluating the association of saturated fat with cardiovascular disease. - 2010
   a. Siri-Tarino, P.W. et al., 2010.
   b. The American Journal of Clinical Nutrition, 91(3), pp.535–546.

    c. Available at:
http://ajcn.nutrition.org/content/
91/3/535

4) Ketogenic diet slows down mitochondrial myopathy progression in mice. - 2010
    a. Ahola-Erkkilä, S. et al., 2010.
    b. Human Molecular Genetics, 19(10), pp.1974–1984.
    c. Available at:
http://hmg.oxfordjournals.org/co
ntent/19/10/1974

5) Effect of low-calorie versus low-carbohydrate ketogenic diet in type 2 diabetes. - 2012
    a. Hussain, T.A. et al., 2012.
    b. Nutrition, 28(10), pp.1016–1021.
    c. Available at:
http://www.nutritionjrnl.com/arti
cle/S0899-9007(12)00073-
1/abstract

6) Ketogenic diet reduces cytochrome c release and cellular apoptosis following traumatic brain injury in juvenile rats - 2009
    a. Hu, Z.G. et al., 2009.
    b. Annals of clinical and laboratory science, 39(1), pp.76–83.

    c. Available at:
http://www.ncbi.nlm.nih.gov/pub
med/19201746

7) Renal function following long-term
weight loss in individuals with
abdominal obesity on a very-low-
carbohydrate diet vs high-carbohydrate
diet. - 2010
    a. Brinkworth, G.D. et al., 2010.
    b. Journal of the American Dietetic
Association, 110(4), pp.633–638.
    c. Available at:
http://www.ncbi.nlm.nih.gov/pub
med/20071648

8) Meta-analysis of prospective cohort
studies evaluating the association of
saturated fat with cardiovascular
disease. - 2010
    a. Siri-Tarino, P.W. et al., 2010.
    b. The American journal of clinical
nutrition, 91(3), pp.535–546.
    c. Available at:
http://www.ncbi.nlm.nih.gov/pub
med/20071648

9) Carbohydrate Restriction has a More
Favorable Impact on the Metabolic
Syndrome than a Low Fat Diet. - 2009
    a. Volek, J.S. et al., 2009.

   b. Lipids, 44(4), pp.297–309.
   c. Available at:
      http://link.springer.com/article/10.100
      7/s11745-008-3274-2

10)   Resistance training in overweight
   women on a ketogenic diet conserved
   lean body mass while reducing body fat.
   - 2010
   a. Jabekk, P.T. et al., 2010.
   b. Nutrition & Metabolism, 7(1), p.17.
   c. Available at:
      http://www.nutritionandmetabolism.c
      om/content/7/1/17/abstract

www.ingramcontent.com/pod-product-compliance
Lightning Source LLC
Chambersburg PA
CBHW071357280526
45787CB00001B/359